YOUR FAT CAN MAKE YOU THIN

Also by Calvin Ezrin, M.D.:

The Type 2 Diabetes Diet Book
(with Robert E. Kowalski)

YOUR FAT CAN MAKE YOU THIN

**The Revolutionary Weight-Loss Program
That Turns Your Body into a
Fat-Burning Machine**

Calvin Ezrin, M.D.

with Kristen L. Caron, M.A.

Foreword by Robert E. Kowalski

CB

CONTEMPORARY BOOKS

Chicago   New York   San Francisco   Lisbon   Madrid   Mexico City   Milan
New Delhi   San Juan   Seoul   Singapore   Sydney   Toronto

The *McGraw-Hill* Companies

Library of Congress Cataloging-in-Publication Data

Ezrin, Calvin.
    Your fat can make you thin : the revolutionary weight-loss program that turns your body into a fat-burning machine / Calvin Ezrin, with Kristen L. Caron ; foreword by Robert E. Kowalski.
        p.   cm.
    Includes bibliographical references and index.
    ISBN 0-7373-0576-2
    1. Low-carbohydrate diet.   2. Reducing diets.   I. Caron, Kristen L.   II. Title.

RM237.73 .E97   2000
613.2'5—dc21   99-087671

    5 6 7 8 9 10 11   DOC/DOC   2 1 0 9 8 7 6 5

ISBN 0-7373-0576-2

Interior design by Robert S. Tinnon

McGraw-Hill books are available at special quantity discounts to use as premiums and sales promotions, or for use in corporate training programs. For more information, please write to the Director of Special Sales, Professional Publishing, McGraw-Hill, Two Penn Plaza, New York, NY 10121-2298. Or contact your local bookstore.

The purpose of this book is to educate. It is sold with the understanding that the publisher and author shall have neither liability nor responsibility for any injury caused or alleged to be caused directly or indirectly by the information contained in this book. While every effort has been made to ensure its accuracy, the book's contents should not be construed as medical advice. Each person's health needs are unique. To obtain recommendations appropriate to your particular situation, please consult a qualified health care provider.

This book is printed on acid-free paper.

This work is dedicated to Gerry (Geraldine),
an outstanding wife and mother of eight,
who has been an inspiration in all my endeavors.

Contents

Foreword by Robert E. Kowalski

xi

Acknowledgments

xv

Prologue

xvii

Part I
THE INSULIN CONTROL DIET

Chapter 1
Your Fat Can Make You Thin

3

Chapter 2
Health Hazards Associated with Obesity

17

Chapter 3
Obesity: A National Problem

31

Chapter 4
Ketosis

35

Chapter 5
Desperately Seeking Serotonin

45

CONTENTS

Chapter 6
The Ins and Outs of Salt and Water
51

Chapter 7
Diabesity: The Link Between Obesity and Diabetes
57

Chapter 8
How to Be Your Own Weight-Loss Doctor
63

Part II
CLIMB ABOARD THE KETOSIS EXPRESS

Chapter 9
Just the Facts: Your Guide to Basic Nutrition
71

Chapter 10
How to Succeed Immediately:
The 1,000-Calorie, 35-Gram Carbohydrate Solution
83

Chapter 11
Support Strategies
103

Chapter 12
Exercise:
The Benefits of Aerobic and Resistance Activity
119

Chapter 13
Beyond Ketosis: Stabilization and Maintenance
129

Chapter 14
Doctor to Doctor:
An Overview of Endocrinology
141

Appendix A
Recipes
141

Appendix B
Food Composition Tables
189

Appendix C
Shopping Lists
223

Bibliography
225

Index
229

Foreword

AT FIRST GLANCE, THIS BOOK MAY seem similar to other diet books on the market, especially those taking a low-carbohydrate approach. But there are vital differences that ultimately can and will result in your success, rather than yet another failure, in attaining and maintaining your goal of a healthy weight.

These differences come down to the credentials and capabilities of the author, Dr. Calvin Ezrin, and to the essential concept of developing good habits rather than bad ones during the weight-loss period. More on that in a bit—but first let me tell you about Dr. Ezrin.

Cal and I have known each other personally and professionally since 1986. You learn a lot about a person in that much time. He is an internationally acclaimed physician and endocrinologist, and one of our greatest authorities on the functional structure of the pituitary gland. Why should you care about that?

Because, in a very real sense, by reading this book and following its program, you are choosing him as *your* physician; and as such, you obviously want the very best. Having exposure and access to doctors across the country in every possible specialty, thanks to the nature of my career as a medical journalist, I confidently refer literally everyone I know and meet who needs weight control to Dr. Ezrin. Aside from being capable and respected, Dr. Ezrin truly cares about his patients.

In contrast to many in our unfortunate era of cynicism and opportunism, you will not find Dr. Ezrin touting and hyping his own products or engaging in self-promotion. He chooses, rather, to spend his time preserving his passion for scientific research within the confines of his medical practice. As such, the advice you are about to receive is based on the most up-to-date medical and scientific thinking and knowledge. Since Dr. Ezrin would doubtless be too modest to actually say so, let me state that the true reason he has written this book is his sense of mission to improve the world's health. He would really rather, if it were at all possible, personally speak with, examine, and treat every single man and woman who has struggled futilely with his or her weight. Since that is obviously not possible, his book becomes the next best thing, an extension of himself. Consider yourself privileged to have him as your doctor.

The second major difference about this book is the very philosophy of its approach. Dr. Ezrin refuses, absolutely refuses, to take the easy route to a bestseller by telling you lies that you can "eat everything you want, never exercise, and lose all the weight you desire." That technique may sell books, but it doesn't serve your health and well-being.

Step by step, you will be learning the good habits that will enable you to lose weight rapidly and start feeling better and happier than you have in years. I know that's true; I've seen it happen time and time again. I don't wish to disparage other diet-book doctors, but it is unconscionable to tell people to consume vast quantities of harmful fat, or to buy and take "specially formulated" supplements, or to rely on food products that have no value other than to expand the author's bank account.

Best of all, as you follow Dr. Ezrin's rock-solid advice, you can expect some pretty spectacular results. You'll sleep better and more restfully. You'll have far more energy. You'll be happier and more content. And you'll lose weight in a rapid and very satisfying manner. Most important, you'll be able to maintain that weight loss permanently.

Throughout the process, you'll come to understand how your body functions, and why it has been, to this point in time, literally working against you. It will be a learning process, and as with any education, you'll be expected to fully participate. For example, you'll be learning a lot of new words and concepts. Things such as the double-edged sword of the hormone insulin and the neurotransmitter serotonin; foreign-sounding words such as TNF-alpha. But don't be discouraged. You've learned new words and ideas before; it wasn't too long ago that the terms *osteoporosis* and *cholesterol* were limited to medical journals.

I know how important it is to take control of one's own health and destiny. I, myself, have borne the cross of heart disease, having suffered a heart attack and two bypass surgeries before the age of forty-one. And I know the absolute joy of having defeated that disease so that I can expect a long life. But that's another story, and the subject of my own books.

On a professional level, it happens that throughout my more than three decades of journalism on health, I've written extensively about weight problems and the frequently accompanying affliction of diabetes. But until I learned about Dr. Ezrin's unique approach, I had never come close to feeling that there truly is an ultimate solution to weight control.

When I first heard Dr. Ezrin's theories, they made scientific sense to me; but the true drama came in meeting the many men and women who have enjoyed spectacular success because Dr. Ezrin was their doctor. And now, he is yours as well. Congratulations!

ROBERT E. KOWALSKI,
author of
The 8-Week Cholesterol Cure

Acknowledgments

OUR SINCEREST THANKS TO AARON HENRY, whose formidable writing skill helped to adorn this work with a sense of style. He transformed an initially unappetizing offering into what we hope will be experienced as a delicious gourmet meal.

We would like to recognize many individuals who have been an integral part of the process of compiling this book. Above all, we would like to thank our families and friends for their unwavering support. Thank you, L. Hudson Perigo, our editor, whose guidance has been indispensable in the creation of this book. Many thanks to Carole Willcocks, whose generosity has been a tremendous gift; our angel, Sue Okuyama, for offering her time and energy; and Dr. Katrina Wood and Corinne Gelfan of Wilshire Counseling Center and Valley Therapy Center for their patience and support.

We would also like to express our gratitude to several patients who offered their time to this project. Their insights have proven invaluable. Thanks to Bea Dinerman, Judson Laff, Shirley Miller, Kari Grubin, Marge Goldblat, Sue Shatzkin, Claire Appruzzi, Barbara Alexander, Michelle Amott, Craig Kirkpatrick, Joyce Kovelman, Carmela Santana, and Priscilla Chirchick.

Prologue

MANY DIET BOOKS HAVE BEEN PRODUCED by writers of questionable authority and credibility, and have initially sold very well—but few have stood the test of time and the impartial experience of others. Legitimate medical investigators who write credibly about the complex factors that control weight gain and loss are wary of recommending simplistic treatment programs that do not have a statistically established, long-term, generally favorable outcome. My present views were shaped in a career that combined clinical (patient-related) and basic research within the practice of endocrinology in an academic, and later a community, setting. My first publication, *Childhood Diabetes*, was written in 1948, the year before I graduated from the University of Toronto Medical School. It began as an oral presentation to the medical faculty—part of an induction process admitting me to Alpha Omega Alpha, a medical honor society analogous to Phi Beta Kappa. In the audience was professor of physiology Dr. Charles Best, the codiscoverer of insulin, who later invited me to do research with him after graduation. At that time, I was also being taught about clinical diabetes by Dr. Robert Kerr, who had been associated in London, England, with Professor Harold Himsworth. Professor Himsworth was the first to suggest that there are two types of diabetes—one insulin sensitive, and the other more resistant to insulin. In retrospect, I realize the great privilege afforded me to be exposed to these giants in the field of diabetes. Their influence had a lasting effect on my career, during which I have never lost touch with the problems of diabetes.

In my postgraduate years, my most influential mentor and role model was Professor Ray Farquharson, chairman of the

Department of Medicine at the University of Toronto and founder of the Medical Research Council of Canada. He was an inspiring lecturer, imparting to medical students the importance of respecting the patient as a sensitive person whose emotions must always be considered in assessing and treating illness.

After graduation, I had planned to train in pediatrics at the world-renowned Hospital for Sick Children in Toronto. First, I had to complete a year called Junior Rotating Internship at the Toronto General Hospital to obtain additional experience in specialties and in medicine and surgery. In the course of this internship, I was asked to see Professor Farquharson about a delicate matter. At this meeting, he admitted that at the University of Toronto there existed a policy of genteel anti-Semitism, which had prevented the appointment of any Jewish physicians to the permanent staff of the university Department of Medicine and the university hospitals. He wanted to change this policy and asked me to consider abandoning my career in pediatrics in favor of one in adult medicine with an emphasis on diabetes and endocrinology. Without hesitation, I accepted.

The next year was spent honoring my commitment to the Hospital for Sick Children, during which time I cared for many children with diabetes. Each diabetic child reminded me of the miracle of insulin. Had it been thirty years or more earlier, not one of these little lives would have been spared. It was a long time before I could consider that insulin, this life-saving angel of mercy, could also have a demonic side, greatly contributing to our present epidemic of increasing obesity.

Following my service at the Hospital for Sick Children, I embarked on thirty-five years of research, beginning with investigations into the endocrine system at the Banting Institute. (The institute was named after the discoverer of insulin, Dr. Fred Banting, who was killed in a plane crash in 1941 while on active service during World War II.) My first task was to investigate the structure and function of the pituitary—or master—gland, which until then had been a mystery. Before long, using differential staining techniques, the cells of origin of the various pituitary hormones were defined. This differentiation of the various cell types was incorporated into standard descriptions and teaching, and later formed the basis of an internationally accepted classification of pituitary tumors. Working in the Banting Institute gave me an inspiring connection with Dr. Banting's aims in medical research. In this setting, I felt that I was linked with both of the discoverers of insulin, Banting and Best, which further solidified my desire to pursue the expanding role of insulin in health and disease. My understanding of the relationship between insulin resistance and obesity led me to formulate the approach to weight loss described in this book.

CALVIN EZRIN, M.D.

PART I

THE INSULIN CONTROL DIET

CHAPTER 1

Your Fat Can Make You Thin

DIETING IS ALWAYS A DIFFICULT PROCESS. It requires behavioral changes, abstaining from foods that give you pleasure, and, despite the support you may enjoy from your family and friends, journeying along a road you ultimately must travel alone. Perhaps the worst aspect of dieting is the probability of failure, as only a small fraction of dieters successfully keep off the weight they have lost. You may have suffered disappointment and the feelings of inadequacy that accompany such failure because, despite the difficult adjustments you made, you ended up at the point where you began. It's important for you to recognize that, in most cases, this failure is not your fault. The weight-loss solutions you've been offered previously require near-impossible tasks. No one can limit himself to a high-fat diet for the rest of his life, forever take appetite suppressants, or subsist entirely on powdered food. But there is a solution.

WHY THE INSULIN CONTROL DIET IS DIFFERENT

The treatment in this book is designed to break the cycle in which you have been trapped. I call the program "The Insulin Control Diet." It has been developed through years of research in endocrinology and has been tried and proven successful with numerous patients in a clinical setting. In its initial phase, the diet will allow you to quickly and safely reach your ideal weight. The next phase will allow you to maintain that weight permanently and without drastic dietary changes from normal. With a few key adjustments in your diet and the introduction of aerobic exercise, you will be able to live your life a changed person, both lightened and enlightened.

I am confident that the diet will work as promised if you follow it as prescribed.

WHAT IS OBESITY?

One useful rule of thumb when approximating ideal body weight for men is to give 110 pounds for the first 5 feet of height and 5 pounds for each additional inch in height above 5 feet, plus or minus 10 percent according to frame size. The rule for women is 100 pounds for the first 5 feet and 5 pounds per additional inch, with the same adjustment for frame size. Medically speaking, anyone whose body weight is over 20 percent above the ideal is considered obese. Anyone whose weight is more than 10 percent above the ideal should be considered overweight.

HOW DOES OBESITY TAKE HOLD OF YOUR LIFE?

There are a variety of hereditary, behavioral, and environmental influences that contribute significantly to weight gain. Many patients tell me that their weight gain began when they stopped smoking. Others blame it on depression. Often, it begins in—and following—pregnancy. Reduced activity may result from painful arthritis; an inability to exercise can also result in added weight. Whatever the initial causes of obesity, the condition itself is not corrected through traditional "dieting."

TRADITIONAL TREATMENTS OF OBESITY

Low-carbohydrate diets are not new, but they have recently experienced a resurgence of popularity. One hundred and fifty years ago in London, England, a cabinetmaker named William Banting (who was a cousin of the ancestors of Frederick Banting, the discoverer of insulin), published a communication entitled *Letter on Corpulence* recommending a low-carbohydrate intake to treat obesity. The idea caught on and has been preserved to the present day. The English still refer to going on a low-carbohydrate modified fast as "doing a Banting." Subsequently, beginning in the mid-twentieth century, the low-carbohydrate idea was revived by Drs. Pennington, Stillman, Tarnower, and, more persistently, Dr. Robert Atkins.

Dr. Atkins has continued to be prominent in this field. His program, since it is so popular, deserves respectful attention. He should be credited with continuing to promote the idea that carbohydrate-induced insulin secretion is harmful to overweight people. He draws the most ire from his critics, however, by asserting that fat need not be restricted in his program. There are three reasons for this criticism. The first is that the extra fat will, in susceptible individuals, contribute to an increase in circulating and tissue cholesterol. This can occur on such a program, but not invariably. In some patients with high cholesterol levels, the major source of this increase is overproduction of cholesterol by the liver, with a relatively minor contribution from dietary cholesterol or saturated fat (which the body turns into cholesterol). If sufficient weight loss is achieved on this program, some patients show decreased cholesterol, reflecting their diminished internal production of this material. Assessing the initial cholesterol status and periodically reevaluating it should settle this question in any given case.

The second issue under contention is whether the extra calories that come from calorie-dense fat significantly interfere with the body's ability to utilize its own fat for energy. I believe this is true, and it is probably the most compelling reason not to add fat to low-carbohydrate programs. Reducing fat in the diet, along with carbohydrate, eliminates concerns about possible harmful effects on the cholesterol level and thereby deals with both of the first two objections.

The third objection is related to the safety of *ketosis,* an induced process of fat burning which is a feature of the Atkins diet. In our chapter on ketosis, we will distinguish between mild, beneficial ketosis and harmful, life-threatening ketosis in uncontrolled diabetes. Mild ketosis cuts the appetite, rids the body of salt and water, and calms the brain. The next level of intensity in controlling hunger we call *anorexia* (not to be confused with the psychological condition *anorexia nervosa*), and extreme ketosis can result in *nausea,* which often leads quickly to vomiting. With the Insulin Control Diet you will maintain a very mild degree of ketosis, in which stored fat is the main source of energy.

The Opti-Fast dietary program was made famous by Oprah Winfrey, who achieved an initially spectacular weight loss that she proudly displayed to the world. Opti-Fast is a convenient powdered form of a low-calorie, low-fat, low-carbohydrate diet with adequate amounts of first-class protein to meet the essential needs of the body, which cannot be supplied by internal processes. Another diet, which was similar but composed of a low-quality protein derived from animal skin (collagen), was responsible for many deaths—mainly from cardiac complications—when it was introduced as the Last Chance Diet about forty years ago. Because there is little or no experience with regular food during the weight-loss phase of the Opti-Fast diet, it is hard for people to adjust to a pattern of normal eating in the maintenance phase; therefore, the long-term results are dismal, with a failure rate of at least 90 percent.

Weight Watchers, an old standby, stresses calorie reduction and increased exercise, with an emphasis on support groups and camaraderie. The results are not impressive, and ultimately, many dieters become discontented and seek help elsewhere.

Jenny Craig and NutriSystem offer packaged food with a structured program of eating based on measured amounts. A substantial support system helps clients to stay on track. What is missing is the exercise of free will and the knowledge to proceed independently after sufficient weight has been lost.

The Lindora program, which features a low-carbohydrate diet and ketone testing (testing for the energy internally produced by ketosis), has the additional feature of regular injections of vitamin B_{12}. At first, Lindora utilized human chorionic gonadotropin (HCG), a pregnancy hormone, mimicking closely the action of a pituitary ovary-stimulating hormone. On the mistaken assumption that HCG had fat-mobilizing power, it was administered widely in weight-loss programs throughout the world. Not long ago in California, a physician was disciplined, based on my testimony, by the attorney general's office for the inappropriate use of HCG injections in weight-loss clinics. As a result of this decision, Lindora discontinued its use of HCG nationally in favor of vitamin B_{12}— which has little obvious therapeutic effect. The major benefit of the injections appears to be the continuing contact with a support staff and the encouragement this undoubtedly provides.

Diet Pills

A discussion of appetite-controlling pills should begin with consideration of phen-fen, which consists of two drugs: phentermine and fenfluramine. This combination provided impressive reduction in food intake, which neither alone could achieve. Phentermine is in the amphetamine family; it stimulates the central nervous sympathetic (adrenaline like) activity, but with fewer side effects. Fenfluramine acts to increase brain serotonin by a combination of inhibiting its reuptake inactivation plus an increased release of serotonin itself. This excess serotonin appears to cause damage to heart valves and, in rare instances, high blood pressure in the pulmonary (lung) arteries. With recognition of these toxic side effects, fenfluramine was withdrawn. Since then, phentermine continues to be used alone. A new agent that inhibits reuptake of both serotonin and norepinephrine (sibutramine, Meridia) has been introduced and appears to be working well to control appetite in most cases, albeit with the additional hazard of aggravating high blood pressure.

Herbal Remedies

Herbal preparations that are advertised to control appetite, increase energy, and elevate mood, and that offer a host of other health and longevity-enhancing benefits, should not be assumed to be beneficial or even harmless. They often contain stimulants, such as ephedra or ma huang, that have adrenaline like qualities. These can be harmful to sensitive individuals—especially those who are hypersensitive to begin with.

WHY DIETS DON'T WORK

If you are overweight, why can't you just reduce your food intake until your surplus fat is shed, and then, to prevent excessive weight loss, resume normal eating? Why can't you just "exercise control"? You know it doesn't work that way. Even if much weight is lost by sustained calorie deficit, the long-term results are dismal. The frequent failure to maintain a significant weight loss has been explained by a "set-point" theory, which maintains that the body works to return to the preestablished higher weight because of an altered metabolism that combats the attempt to be thinner. There is no hard evidence for this, although it is intellectually appealing. Regardless, one year after goal weight is achieved, only 10 to 20 percent of dieters are able to maintain it. Most of the "regainers" return to their starting weights, and sometimes they gain even more than that. This is because traditional diet plans fail to address the metabolic consequences of obesity.

METABOLISM
AND THE ROLE OF INSULIN

The first metabolic consequence involves the role of the hormone insulin, a substance known to most Americans but understood by few. Simply put, insulin spurs the process by which glucose (blood sugar) in the blood is allowed to enter the cells, where it can be used for energy. Without insulin, blood sugar builds to dangerous levels. Most people know that diabetics, who lack insulin or have inadequate amounts, must compensate with medical treatment. But what is not widely known is that metabolically, diabetes and obesity are closely linked—a relationship we will explain more fully in chapter 7, "Diabesity." For now, we will focus on answering the question, Why can't you lose weight merely by reducing food intake?

A major reason why this scenario doesn't work is insulin resistance, which accompanies weight gain and increases along with it. If you gain as little as 20 pounds of weight, for whatever reason, that extra fat produces a chemical that selectively blocks the blood sugar–lowering effect of insulin. This antagonist is called TNF-alpha (tumor necrosis factor alpha). Originally we thought TNF-alpha was simply a localized cell-to-cell communicator. Now we know that it also travels in the bloodstream as a hormone; and it is in this capacity that it influences insulin. Insulin has three major functions: to lower blood sugar, to build up fat, and to retain salt and water. In fat tissue, TNF-alpha acts both as a hormone and as a "hormone antagonist," preventing insulin from breaking down your blood sugar. As a result, the blood sugar level rises, stimulating the secretion of more insulin to restore the blood sugar to normal. But even if your blood sugar is measured at that time and remains normal, your metabolism may still be fighting against you, via the excess of insulin.

Remember that insulin is not only the blood sugar–lowering hormone; it is also the fat-building and fat-storing hormone, functions that are not affected by TNF-alpha. Excess insulin builds fat by increasing your appetite, particularly for carbohydrates. This extra fat produces more TNF-alpha, which in turn results in more insulin and more weight gain. I call this sequence the "Metabolic Trap of Obesity."

Even if you reduce your food intake, the Metabolic Trap of Obesity may hinder you in losing weight. More important, without regulating your diet to make sure that you are eating the *right* foods, the *types* of foods you eat may maintain your weight and even increase it. And so, the Metabolic Trap of Obesity becomes a vicious cycle. Fortunately, it can be broken with the Insulin Control Diet.

While the initial causes of weight gain should not be ignored (e.g., changes in your diet, lifestyle, or medication), these are not nearly as important as recognizing that excess insulin (hyperinsulinism) is the major driving force for the persistence and, likely, worsening of your obesity. With these processes in mind, we come to the first step in the solution: You can reduce your insulin with a *low-carbohydrate, low-calorie diet,* supplemented by *aerobic exercise.*

Only by reducing your insulin can fat escape from storage to become a major source of energy and a beneficial "natural pharmacy," whereby your appetite is reduced and salt and water are eliminated, as if you were using prescription drugs, but without their potential hazards. Once the fat is released by lowering insulin, your body will begin to internally consume calories and your hunger for external calories will decrease. In this way, *your fat will make you thin.*

The reduction of calories and carbohydrates (which lowers your insulin) makes dieting easy, with quick weight loss and little or no hunger. Reducing diets that *do not* restrict carbohydrates are harder to follow because hunger is not well controlled. Even the addition of a relatively safe diet pill, which helps achieve initial success, does not improve the long-term outcome. Such medication must be continued indefinitely—with still-uncertain consequences.

METABOLISM AND THE ROLE OF SEROTONIN

The second metabolic consequence of dieting involves a brain chemical called *serotonin.* Your brain is composed of billions of nerve cells (neurons) which are like elongated electrical wires.

Unlike electrical wires, however, which communicate by direct contact with each other, nerve cells are separated by gaps (synapses) that have to be bridged by chemical messengers called neuro transmitters.

Serotonin (which will be discussed more thoroughly in chapter 5) is the most important of the forty known neurotransmitters in the regulation of both appetite and sleep. It's helpful to imagine serotonin as being stored in a reservoir in the brain. Normally, the body replenishes it through deep, restorative sleep; however, some serotonin is required initially at the onset of sleep to achieve a good night's rest.

Carbohydrates, by stimulating insulin production, can boost serotonin levels, but only temporarily. Deficiency of serotonin produces carbohydrate cravings; when you satisfy these cravings with carbohydrates, more serotonin is made from the increase of insulin that follows. Some carbohydrates, notably chocolate, have come to be known as "comfort food" because of the calming effect of increased serotonin. This contentment is short lived, however, usually lasting less than an hour or two. Despite the fleeting pleasure you may derive from comfort food, the increased calories you ingest will remain. Along with the salt and water retention induced by insulin, these calories contribute to a rapid and alarming gain in weight.

Serotonin cannot be measured in blood tests because it is too big to pass through the "curtain" that separates the brain from the bloodstream (the blood/brain barrier). Nevertheless, when there are carbohydrate cravings and sleep disturbances with a lack of daytime energy, we can conclude that serotonin is lacking.

Stress also affects serotonin. Increased stress triggers the demand for *more* serotonin, but *less* is produced because stress also interferes with deep, restorative sleep—essential to the natural production of the chemical. Patients struggling to maintain weight after a considerable loss are almost invariably serotonin-depleted. In this setting, no "diet" can succeed.

WHAT, THEN, IS THE SOLUTION?

Controlling the levels of insulin and serotonin are the primary considerations in successfully achieving weight loss. A lack of serotonin is the best explanation for the nearly inevitable relapse that accompanies attempts at maintenance; so some form of serotonin enhancement, either at the beginning of, during, or after weight loss, may be necessary to maintain your weight goals.

Other low-carbohydrate, low-calorie diets have not previously addressed this critical problem, but I recommend the prescription drug trazodone (a serotonin enhancer) to help you achieve a state of deep, energizing sleep. The dosage of trazodone used in this diet is *very much lower* than the dosage used for trazodone's original antidepressant usage (see page **46**). Still, a physician must oversee your program to monitor your usage of trazodone. Most, but not all, patients require the use of trazodone during the diet; however, the medication is temporary. After you achieve your goal weight, your serotonin levels should be adequately restored and you should no longer need the help of medication. However, the amount of time each individual patient uses trazodone varies. When you begin to reintroduce carbohydrate into your diet after the weight-loss phase, you may gradually withdraw trazodone.

Once sufficient serotonin is provided to produce an improved sleep pattern, which may take only two or three nights, the second step of my diet plan is to control your insulin levels; this will bring about sustained weight loss. This strategy works even when the cause of the original weight gain cannot be eliminated. For example, many medications used in psychiatry unfortunately lead to weight gain. If used early enough, the Insulin Control Diet can prevent such gain, and when obesity has already occurred, the Insulin Control Diet can still achieve results even if you continue to take psychiatric medication.

The Greeks had a word, *panacea,* which means a "cure or control of all ills." Applied to the growing problem of obesity in our society, the Insulin Control Diet qualifies as a panacea, a control of all the ills associated with obesity.

In the following pages you will learn the details of our program for success. On page 15 is a typical case study from my practice, illustrating many of the points we've made in this chapter.

In the chapters that follow, we describe the details of the weight-loss phase and the transition through stabilization to the lifelong maintenance that is the expected outcome of our program. Join us in a journey that will change your life.

A ROAD MAP TO "YOUR FAT WILL MAKE YOU THIN"

This book is divided into two sections. In the early chapters of the first section, we provide descriptions of the terms that are key components in the process of the Insulin Control Diet: ketosis, insulin, and serotonin.

The second section, "Climb Aboard the Ketosis Express," is devoted to the easy application of the principles to your diet in order to achieve a state of ketosis (fat burning), in which you will be able to achieve your weight-loss goals. We will provide menus, recipes, and support strategies to keep you focused. In addition, the second section deals with stabilization and maintenance of your weight. This is a crucial stage in your diet. Unlike other diets,

---

• CASE STUDY •

Susan was thirty-seven years of age, 5 feet, 5 inches tall, and weighed over 200 pounds. She told me that when she married at age twenty-five, her weight was 130 pounds. With her first pregnancy at age twenty-seven, she gained 50 pounds and delivered a 9-pound baby. She kept 30 of these extra pounds after her first pregnancy and added another 30 pounds after she had her second child at age thirty-two. During the second pregnancy, she developed gestational diabetes (pregnancy-related diabetes) in the last three months, which required insulin for control until after delivery, when it disappeared. Diet, exercise, and even appetite pills didn't work for her. She retained fluid easily, particularly after ingesting carbohydrates. She also had trouble falling asleep; she woke easily during the night and felt tired in the morning. By the middle of the afternoon, she was ready for a nap, and then even after dinner she had no energy to go out.

After the delivery of Susan's second child, the pregnancy hormones that interfered with insulin's blood sugar–lowering effect were eliminated. She still had the potential for diabetes, which might well have developed if she had continued to gain weight. In order to lose weight, she had to reduce her need for insulin. A low-carbohydrate diet plus aerobic exercise is the best way to achieve this. I explained to her the way in which fat is held in storage until released by decreasing insulin levels. When liberated rapidly, the fat would become her body's main source of energy, serving as a "high-octane" fuel for muscles, the brain, and all other organs. It would become a "beneficial natural pharmacy" as well, capable of providing excellent appetite control, salt and water elimination, and a calming effect on her brain. I explained also that medication at bedtime would improve her sleep and produce a small amount of supplemental serotonin; deep sleep would in turn replenish her brain's store of this important chemical. Finally, Susan was given details about diet and exercise.

---

which can—and most often do—lead to relapse, our program makes it easy for you to reach your weight goals and stay there. This requires a continuing awareness of your diet and the important inclusion of exercise activities in your weekly schedule. Ultimately, your success will be rewarded with health, energy, longevity, happiness, and an improved self-image.

FINALLY, A WORD ABOUT EXERCISE

Whatever diet recommendations are made, everyone agrees that increased exercise should be an important part of the package. Much obesity is the result of an inability to exercise because of painful arthritis, neurologic impairment, emotional inhibition, or a failure to acknowledge the necessity for exercise. The importance of exercise cannot be overemphasized, even if it begins with baby steps, and we'll discuss this more completely in subsequent chapters.

SUMMARY

- The Insulin Control Diet allows you to lose weight and keep it off through a ketogenic, low-carbohydrate, low-calorie diet and aerobic exercise.
- Control of serotonin and insulin in your body is key to the diet.
- Programs that do not replenish your serotonin level are almost certainly doomed to fail.

CHAPTER 2

Health Hazards Associated with Obesity

THE MEDICAL RISKS OF OBESITY

BEFORE DISCUSSING THE DIET, I WILL stress the importance of weight loss for obese patients. For your overall well-being, the weight-loss program you embark on should be one that works effectively and safely, and on which you can maintain your goal once you have shed excess weight.

Obesity is associated with many serious medical risks, most of which are, at least in part, reversible with a substantial loss of weight. As you will see from the examples and case studies that follow, the Insulin Control Diet has effectively reversed many medical problems related to obesity in my patients; it is a panacea for the ills of obesity.

Those diseases whose risk is increased by obesity can be classified into two categories. In the first group are risks that result from the metabolic changes associated with excess fat. These include:

- diabetes
- pancreatitis
- high blood pressure (hypertension)
- gallbladder disease

- some forms of cancer that are associated with obesity
- fatty livers
- infertility

The second group of disorders are the result of the increased weight of the fat itself. These include:

- osteoarthritis
- snoring and sleep apnea
- the emotional and social burden of obesity
- proneness to accidents

In addition, and most seriously, obesity is associated with an increased risk of death, as demonstrated in life insurance statistics.

Diabetes

Diabetes will be addressed in detail in chapter 7, "Diabesity."

Pancreatitis

Obesity is often associated with elevated triglycerides and LDL (low-density lipoprotein, or *bad* cholesterol), as well as with HDL (high-density lipoprotein, or *good* cholesterol). With highly elevated triglycerides, there is a strong possibility of acute pancreatitis, a serious abdominal emergency.

High Blood Pressure (Hypertension)

Blood pressure is frequently increased in overweight individuals. Obesity and hypertension conspire to reduce cardiac function, although by somewhat different mechanisms. The hypertension of obesity appears to be related to increased sympathetic activity —the result of hyperinsulinism. Hypertension is strongly associated with Type 2 diabetes and a high blood level of triglycerides and cholesterol. This combination of hypertension and increased triglycerides/cholesterol is sometimes called Syndrome X, or "The Metabolic Syndrome." Obese individuals with body fat mainly in the abdominal area (i.e., apple-shaped obesity) are at a higher risk for diabetes and heart disease then those with pear-shaped obesity, involving mainly the buttocks.

This deadly quartet of obesity, diabetes, hypertension, and hyperlipidemia (elevated lipids, or fat, in the blood) is responsible for a large number of deaths from cardiovascular causes. Experience has shown that it is now necessary to treat all four of these disorders as aggressively as possible; otherwise, the risk of a fatal outcome will remain significant.

Mark was 5 feet, 11 inches tall and weighed 275 pounds, about 100 pounds overweight. He was a high-strung, obese diabetic with high blood pressure that was difficult to control. In spite of taking four differently directed antihypertensive medications, his blood pressure remained dangerously high—170/110. He knew that the combination of diabetes and hypertension is often lethal because of stroke, heart attacks, and kidney failure, alone or in combination. His blood pressure medicines had been chosen carefully, starting with the most logical, an angiotensin-converting enzyme (ACE) inhibitor. This drug blocks the production of angiotensin, one of the most powerful blood pressure–elevating elements in the body; however, its effect was not enough to bring his blood pressure down. Thereafter, he was given a calcium channel blocker, which works in another fashion to limit spasm of the arteries. Because hypertension was still unrelieved, he was given a potassium-sparing diuretic, which sometimes is helpful, but his high blood pressure persisted. Finally, a beta receptor–

blocking drug was given to prevent adrenaline from connecting with its receptors that produce spasm in the artery wall.

Trazodone and the Insulin Control Diet were added to the treatment mix. Instead of the usually recommended 5 grams of salt, because of his hypertension, salt intake was limited to 2 grams and his electrolytes were followed carefully. In one month, he lost 20 pounds and his blood pressure had dropped to 130/85. He was sleeping well, was more relaxed at work, and was not hungry. Over the next four months, as his weight fell further, his blood pressure pills were gradually withdrawn, leaving him with only the ACE inhibitor to maintain his now-normal blood pressure. His diabetes, which was treated only with Glucophage, also showed improvement. His initial glycohemoglobin of 10 percent fell to 6 percent, the upper limit of normal.

It is not unusual for weight loss to lower high blood pressure, although the mechanism remains somewhat controversial. In simple models, insulin's effect on blood pressure is to lower it by relaxing arterial walls; however, hyperinsulinism sensitizes the arterial walls to adrenaline. Insulin also promotes retention of salt and water, which aggravates hypertension. Reducing these influences through weight loss can then lower blood pressure. Weight loss is very helpful in treating obese, hypertensive diabetics.

Gallbladder Disease

Gallbladder disease, which involves the formation of gallstones, is strongly associated with being overweight. The increased risk of gallstones is related to the fact that internal cholesterol production is increased with significant weight gain; and it appears to be derived directly from body fat. This increased cholesterol is excreted in the bile, or is likely to be precipitated into gallstones in the gallbladder. During weight loss, there is also an increased chance of gallstone formation because the released cholesterol is excreted through the bile ducts. Diets with moderate levels of fat, such as the Insulin Control Diet, trigger gallbladder contractions that are sufficient to empty the gallbladder of bile, but not vigorous enough to dislodge any gallstones it may contain.

Cancer

The risk of cancers of the breast, uterus, colon, and prostate are also increased by obesity, presumably because of the cell-stimulating influence of hyperinsulinism (excess insulin in the blood).

Fatty Livers

Obese patients often have fatty livers, likely the result of hyperinsulinism, which stimulates increased liver production of triglycerides, a storage form of fat. The liver, which ordinarily detoxifies substances in the body, performs poorly when it becomes fatty.

Gerald, age forty-five, was an obese alcoholic. He was 5 feet, 5 inches tall and weighed 200 pounds. Ashamed of himself, he had tried to stop drinking abruptly and developed delirium tremens (DTs) with associated convulsions that brought him to the hospital emergency room. His liver function tests, which had been normal a year before, were now moderately elevated, but he was not yet a diabetic.

When I examined him there was no jaundice, but his liver edge could be felt slightly below the rib margin, so it was fair to assume that he had a fatty liver brought on by his alcoholism. This condition would likely go on to cause sufficient scarring (cirrhosis) to produce liver failure or liver cancer if he did not give up alcohol.

Liver cells are exquisite metabolic machines that make fat (triglycerides), carbohydrates (glucose and glycogen, or animal starch), and several proteins. They are also your body's source of ketones, the breakdown products of fat. Because the liver is also the main detoxification center of the body, it requires a small amount of protective glycogen ("animal starch") to be in storage at all times. Even in the state of ketosis, there is a small but reduced amount of glycogen available to serve this role; however, in the extreme situation of a fatty liver (in which the cells are packed with stored triglyceride), there is not enough glycogen available to protect the cells from toxins. In the month prior to starting the ketogenic Insulin Control Diet, Gerald maintained a normal carbohydrate intake in his diet (as should other patients like him) to enable the liver to replenish its glycogen-protective stores.

Having established that Gerald's liver function tests had returned to normal, he followed the Insulin Control Diet with excellent results—a loss of 3 pounds per week on average.

Infertility

Marie, age thirty-five, had been married for fifteen years but had not been able to get pregnant. Her periods, which began in her midteens, had been irregular, and she would often go as long as three months without one. She was 5 feet, 2 inches tall and weighed 250 pounds. She also complained of acne, facial hair growth, and loss of scalp hair. Blood tests showed features consistent with polycystic ovarian disorder—increased androgens (male hormones) and hyperinsulinism. A pelvic ultrasound confirmed the presence of significant ovarian cysts. Marie was treated with a low-calorie, low-carbohydrate diet to reduce the insulin that was driving her to overproduce androgens from the ovary. She reduced her weight to 170 pounds, losing about 2 pounds per week on average. She planned to lose another 40 pounds before attempting to get pregnant. The less she weighs, within reason, the easier her pregnancy will be and the more likely it will be uncomplicated.

Osteoarthritis

The most important arthritic consequence of obesity is osteoarthritis, which is significantly increased in overweight individuals. It most seriously affects the knees and hips, and may be aggravated by the mechanical stress produced by the excess body weight. Osteoarthritis is responsible for a great deal of the disability associated with obesity.

Bob was a fifty-five-year-old retired businessman who was referred to me by his rheumatologist because of resistant obesity of many years' duration that was stressing his hips. He was scheduled for a left hip replacement because of severe degeneration of the cartilage from osteoarthritis, and he wanted to know if there was any way to avoid surgery. He was 5 feet, 8 inches tall and weighed 250 pounds. When he married at age twenty-five, he weighed 160 pounds. After he stopped smoking at age thirty, he started to gain weight and continued to do so in spite of his best efforts. He was particularly fond of warm bread and rolls, a liking that he traced to his grandfather's bakery, which he would visit every morning from his flat upstairs.

On a low-carbohydrate, ketogenic diet with as much structured exercise as his sore hips could tolerate, Bob lost 8 pounds in the first two weeks, and 3 pounds a week steadily thereafter. By the time he reached 200 pounds, his hips felt so much better that surgery was deferred. Subsequently, he reduced to 165 pounds, where he remained with the aid of small doses of trazodone. If he gains as little as 5 pounds, he reinstitutes the ketogenic diet program until he is back to his goal weight.

Sleep Apnea

Sleep apnea (absent breathing) is a potentially lethal condition, as it can lead to cardiac arrest because of prolonged deficiency of oxygen.

Frank, age forty-two, and his wife Henrietta, age thirty-eight, consulted me at the same time about their resistant weight conditions. An additional concern was Frank's snoring and sleep apnea, which had led them to sleep in separate bedrooms. Frank was 6 feet, 1 inch tall and weighed 250 pounds—40 of which he had gained in the past year after some business reverses. He admitted he had uncontrollable carbohydrate cravings. After initial trouble falling asleep, he would snore very loudly and periodically stop breathing for several seconds. This usually caused him to awaken briefly and he would then experience difficulty returning to sleep. In the morning, he was exhausted and sustained himself only with frequent cups of coffee. By the afternoon, he was looking for a place to take a nap, and on the long drive home from work, he found himself almost falling asleep at the wheel. On trazodone and a low-calorie, low-carbohydrate diet, the quality of his sleep improved. He lost weight at a rate of 2½ pounds a week, because he was able to control his carbohydrate cravings. His snoring and sleep apnea disappeared after a loss of 30 pounds. He has normal daytime energy and is in good spirits, having moved back into the family bedroom now that the snoring has ceased.

Henrietta, who weighed 160 pounds at 5 feet, 4 inches tall, lost to her goal weight of 125 at the rate of 2 pounds a week on a similar program of carbohydrate and calorie restriction, plus a small dose of trazodone. Frank and Henrietta felt the support they gave each other was very influential in their mutual success.

Severe Acne

Xenia came to me complaining about the acne breakouts on her face, chest, and back. She also mentioned in passing that she had gained 40 pounds since starting her periods three years before. She was seventeen years of age, 5 feet, 3 inches tall, and weighed 165 pounds. There were no other abnormalities on her physical examination.

In a patient with polycystic ovarian disorder, acne can result from excessive androgen (male hormones), which is linked to insulin; therefore, being overweight can aggravate skin disorders. A blood test revealed that, like Marie, Xenia had increased androgens arising from both the ovaries and the adrenals. These androgens were not in their final active forms; they have to travel to the skin's oil glands (sebaceous glands) to be taken up within the cells, where they are transformed into their final form. Treatment of this condition involved suppressing the adrenals and the ovaries' output of androgens with small doses of safe medications, plus another drug designed to inhibit the activation of the androgens within the skin.

This is a remarkably effective program that brings considerable relief to the acne-ridden patient within a month or so; however, it has to be continued for one to two years in order to be lastingly effective. At the same time, Xenia was treated with a diet low in calories and carbohydrates to help her lose weight while she was dealing with her skin. She was very grateful for the combined improvement and, in particular, for the weight loss of 30 pounds, which she had not anticipated—she had not complained about her weight on her first visit, because she'd felt at the time there was nothing more that could be done.

Massive Obesity

Marvin, a forty-year-old college professor, came to me massively obese. He was 5 feet, 8 inches tall and weighed 450 pounds, a weight he had to use an industrial scale to determine. He was told he had hypoglycemia because his symptoms of anxiety responded promptly to carbohydrate foods. His most rapid, recent weight gain followed the breakup of a relationship, which devastated him. During an anxiety attack, his blood sugar was found to be normal; but at the same time, his blood insulin level was astronomical—twenty times what would be expected in a normal-weight individual. He responded well to a low-calorie, low-carbohydrate diet as well as to trazodone, which has helped to improve the quality of his sleep from a superficial, dream-ridden state to a deeper one that energizes and calms him. His "hypoglycemic" attacks were clearly the result of a lack of serotonin, which could be only temporarily relieved by carbohydrate.

Proneness to Accidents

Beyond the damage that extra weight causes to joints, the chance that an obese person will suffer accidents is greatly increased. A man who weighs twice his ideal weight is twelve times as likely as one at ideal weight to die as a result of an accident.

BODY MASS INDEX: HOW TO KNOW IF YOU'RE OBESE

Physicians, dietitians, and other health professionals now assess weight in terms of body mass index (BMI), a measure of body fat that corrects for height. BMI is derived by dividing weight in kilograms by the square of height in meters. The dividing line between healthy and unhealthy weight is generally accepted to be a BMI of 25. Beyond that point, the risk of heart disease, diabetes, and hypertension climbs rapidly. Another way of determining BMI without using the metric system is the following equation: BMI equals 703 times your weight in pounds divided by your height in inches squared.

$$BMI = \frac{703 \times \text{weight in pounds}}{\text{height in inches}^2}$$

The ideal percentages of body fat for men and women are shown in Table 2.1.

Table 2.1 Body Mass Index (BMI)

Height	Weight				
5' 1"	127	132	137	143	158
5' 2"	131	136	142	147	164
5' 3"	135	141	146	152	169
5' 4"	140	145	151	157	174
5' 5"	144	150	156	162	180
5' 6"	148	150	156	162	186
5' 7"	153	159	166	172	191
5' 8"	158	164	171	177	197
5' 9"	162	169	176	182	203
5' 10"	167	174	181	188	207
5' 11"	172	179	186	193	215
6'	177	184	191	199	221
6' 1"	182	189	197	204	227
BMI	24*	25†	26†	27†	30‡

* BMI of 24 or under: healthy
† BMI of 25–29: overweight
‡ BMI of 30 or more: extremely obese
Source: *The Type 2 Diabetes Diet Book, 3d edition* (Los Angeles: Lowell House, 1999).

There are many charts and tables available which can give you an idea of what may be an ideal body weight for you. One such table is Table 2.2.

In medicine, we often make treatment decisions based on a comparison of the risks and benefits involved. This is called the risk-to-benefit ratio. In treating mild to moderate obesity, there is no doubt that the rewards of successful treatment greatly outweigh the minimal likelihood of any adverse side effects. For more severe or marked obesity, even though the risks are greater, the potential benefit is greater still; the risk-to-benefit ratio is even more favorable, especially in the hands of a knowledgeable physician. Greatly overweight people are in a fragile state of health, but they have much well-being to gain by losing fat.

Table 2.2 Desirable Weights for Men and Women

Height (with shoes)	Weight (with indoor clothing in lbs.)		
	Small Frame	Medium Frame	Large Frame
Men			
5' 2"	112–120	118–129	126–141
5' 3"	115–123	121–133	129–144
5' 4"	118–126	124–136	132–148
5' 5"	121–129	127–139	135–152
5' 6"	124–133	130–143	138–156
5' 7"	128–137	134–147	142–161
5' 8"	132–141	138–152	147–166
5' 9"	136–145	142–156	151–170
5' 10"	140–150	146–160	155–174
5' 11"	144–154	150–165	159–179
6'	148–158	154–170	164–184
6' 1"	152–162	158–175	168–189
6' 2"	156–167	162–180	173–194
6' 3"	160–171	167–185	178–199
6' 4"	164–175	172–190	182–204
Women			
4' 10"	92–98	96–107	104–119
4' 11"	94–101	98–110	106–122
5' 0"	96–104	101–113	109–125
5' 1"	99–107	104–116	112–128
5' 2"	102–110	107–119	115–131
5' 3"	105–113	110–122	118–134
5' 4"	108–116	113–126	121–138
5' 5"	111–119	116–130	125–142
5' 6"	114–123	120–135	129–146
5' 7"	118–127	124–139	133–150
5' 8"	122–131	128–143	137–154
5' 9"	126–135	132–147	141–158
5' 10"	130–140	136–151	145–163
5' 11"	134–144	140–155	149–168
6'	138–148	144–159	153–173

Source: Prepared by the Metropolitan Life Insurance Company. Derived primarily from data of the *Build and Blood Pressure Study,* 1959, Society of Actuaries.

CHAPTER 3

Obesity: A National Problem

WHY IS THERE A NEED FOR ANOTHER DIET BOOK? Because the war against obesity is being lost. One hundred years ago, being over-weight was a relatively rare condition—a luxury accorded mainly to the leisure class. Today, there is an epidemic of increasing proportions in the Western world, with 50 percent of the adult population overweight or obese. If the present trend continues, within twenty years or fewer, more than 75 percent of the population will be significantly obese; that is, more than 20 percent over ideal body weight.

In conjunction with California's Obesity Awareness Month, the American Heart Association released the following obesity statistics:

- More than 50 percent of American children eat too much sugar, fat, and cholesterol.
- Approximately half of these children (25 percent of all American children) are overweight or at risk of being so.
- Up to 20 percent of these overweight children will remain so throughout their lives.
- Being overweight in childhood is the leading cause of pediatric hypertension (high blood pressure in children).

Childhood obesity is only part of the problem in America; in addition:

- Obesity contributes to over 50 percent of the chronic diseases in Western societies.
- Obesity costs an estimated $100 billion nationwide.

What accounts for the $100 billion national cost of obesity?

- Approximately 70 percent of diagnosed cases of cardiovascular disease are related to obesity.
- The average expected lifetime medical care costs for the treatment of heart disease is as much as $6,000 higher for obese patients than for nonobese patients. When these additional expenses per patient are added together, we arrive at the staggering cost of obesity that we all share.

Also contributing to the national problem:

- Approximately 80 percent of patients with Type 2 diabetes are obese.
- Children of obese parents have more than double the risk of becoming obese.

Looking at these statistics, we cannot overstate the magnitude of the problem; obesity is killing us.

An ancient Roman once said, "Gluttony kills more than the sword," showing that obesity was recognized as a health hazard even in the times of the Roman Empire. Today, the health consequences of obesity are becoming well known, with Type 2 diabetes, osteoarthritis, coronary heart disease, hypertension, and gallbladder disease the most prominent. In spite of large public-health expenditures promoting the benefits of exercise and caloric restriction, the incidence of unhealthy weight continues to increase. In recent years, much has been learned about the regulation of appetite and the control of metabolism, but no magic pill has emerged that will permanently control obesity.

In my many years of medical practice, I have discovered that the best treatment for overweight individuals combines control of insulin and of serotonin. The purposes of this book are twofold:

- To share these insights with you, so you may discuss them with your physician.
- To provide the information you need to begin, follow, self-monitor, and maintain a program of permanent weight loss.

From antiquity, the major role of the physician has been to heal the sick. An equally important and more far-reaching obligation is to prevent illness whenever possible. This strikingly effective treatment of overweight individuals by controlling insulin and serotonin can help accomplish both of these aims.

THE EVOLUTION OF OBESITY

Why are we Americans getting fatter faster than the rest of the world? We have adaptive mechanisms that were developed by evolution to favor survival in an environment of uncertain food supply. Now, for the first time in human history, we have food in abundance—so much so, that the few defenses we possess to forestall obesity are overwhelmed. Because of a comparable abundance of food and jobs requiring less exercise, the other countries in the Western world are rapidly catching up to us in the attainment of an obese majority in their populations.

The Pima Indians of the southwest United States are the best-studied Native Americans with regard to the problems of obesity and related Type 2 diabetes. A previously nomadic population, in the present century they have become well fed, with a sedentary lifestyle. Weight gain among the Pima Indians begins early, often in childhood, with frequent pregnancy-related diabetes and large–birth-weight babies. Their genetically related cousins, the Pima Bajos, living in barren Mexican highlands, are forced to work hard with barely adequate food; they have remained lean with a very low incidence of diabetes. From this example, we can see that being overweight and developing diabetes are determined more by lifestyle than genetics.

Apart from the extreme example of the Pima Indians and their cousins, not everybody can become obese. About 25 percent of the human population appears to have a defense against easily gaining fat weight. Simply stated, the more such people eat, the more calories they burn. We are not certain how this happens, but it appears to be, at least in part, related to the "thermogenic" or calorie-burning effect of food, acting through the autonomic or automatic nervous system. Such people also seem to have a more tightly regulated control of their food intake. Signals from relatively minor increases in stored fat probably subtly reduce appetite and increase metabolism in ways that are difficult to measure. The newly discovered hormone leptin, which arises in fat, probably plays a significant role in this adaptation. If only we could all be so fortunate!

Notwithstanding the contribution that these genetic factors make to the problem of obesity, environment—including culture—plays the largest part in determining who will grow fat and who will stay lean. Because of the health hazards of obesity, who will grow fat determines who will die more readily. Over time, a human population will become leaner because of the attrition caused by obesity, but this savage Darwinian mechanism of "survival of the fittest" is not an attractive way to solve our present problem.

CHAPTER 4

Ketosis

WHAT IS KETOSIS?

THE KEY TO UNLOCKING THE METABOLIC TRAP of obesity is the physiological process known as ketosis, in which the liver produces substances called ketones from fatty acids that have been liberated from fat tissue. The process of ketosis, and how to induce it, forms the cornerstone of the first stage of the Insulin Control Diet; therefore, it is important to have some understanding of the process and how it relates to weight loss. In the simplest terms, ketosis results from the rapid burning of fat—using your own fat as a calorie source rather than ingesting calories from food.

Free fatty acids are normally liberated from stored triglycerides (fatty substances circulating in the blood, synthesized from carbohydrate) through exercise; however, this transformation is markedly impaired in obesity because of hyperinsulinism, which inhibits the breakdown of fat.

Exercise lowers blood sugar without involving insulin, thereby decreasing the amount of excess insulin in the blood. Also, because the low-calorie, low-carbohydrate weight-loss diet reduces levels of circulating insulin, free fatty acid liberation is improved. For fat to become the body's major source of energy, the body must use its stored fat as fuel. To allow this process to occur, insulin must be decreased and glucagon (a hormone that drives the production of ketones) must be increased. A substantial restriction of carbohydrate intake achieves both.

The small amount of ketones produced by a low-carbohydrate diet are well tolerated and never induce any disturbance in the normal, slightly alkaline status of the body. Bad ketosis, or ketoacidosis, was the often fatal outcome of uncontrolled diabetes in the preinsulin era. Happily, nowadays it is very rare, occurring only in neglected or unrecognized diabetics with severe insulin deficiency. It is called ketoacidosis because the accompanying massive breakdown of fat produces sufficient ketones and associated fatty acids to make the body more acidic. Diabetic ketoacidosis is invariably associated with high blood sugar in a very sick patient; do not confuse the mild beneficial ketosis of our program with this life-threatening disorder.

FAT: A BENEFICIAL NATURAL PHARMACY

In our culture, fat is unloved. For legitimate medical reasons, as well as cosmetic considerations, most people would rather be at normal weight. Fat, however, has the potential to limit itself if properly directed.

Stored fat consists mainly of triglycerides, which are composed of three fatty acids attached to a glycerol backbone. Triglycerides are derived from three sources: dietary fat, transformation from carbohydrates in the liver, and local manufacture in fat cells. Triglycerides are too big to be released directly into the bloodstream. They must first liberate their fatty acids, which then are available as a major source of energy for all tissues. Insulin, the fat-building and fat-storing hormone in the body, favors the manufacture of triglycerides and interferes with their breakdown.

In addition to triglycerides, fat contains hormones, two of which are very influential in regulating the amount of fat in the body. Leptin is a recently discovered hormone that is made in fat tissue. It was originally described in a strain of mice who, because they lacked this substance, became very obese. When leptin was provided by injection or cross-circulation experiments with normal mice, the obesity was reversed. In humans, leptin's role in obesity is much more complex. Leptin blood levels in obese patients are usually higher than normal, suggesting that resistance to leptin, rather than deficiency, is present. Leptin appears to curb hunger, increase metabolism, and regulate the onset of puberty. At present, it has no role in the treatment of human obesity.

Tumor necrosis factor alpha (TNF-alpha) is a chemical identified originally by its ability, when present in large quantities, to destroy tumor cells. More recently, it has been found in fat tissue and—by sensitive techniques—can be measured in the circulation, where it appears to act as a hormone. In these low amounts, its chief action is to inhibit the blood sugar–lowering effect of insulin. Were it not for a compensatory rise in insulin, the blood sugar would increase to dangerous levels; however, the extra insulin required to control blood sugar leads to more weight gain. The added fat produces more TNF-alpha, which results in further increased insulin.

How easily fat can accumulate! The harm it can do is well known. How can we change fat from an enemy into a friend? By reducing insulin (with a low-carbohydrate diet and aerobic exercise) sufficiently to liberate stored fat rapidly—the process of ketosis. Fat then takes over from carbohydrate as the body's major source of energy. What follows is medical magic. Fat, as it is being utilized as fuel, is converted from an enemy into a beneficial natural pharmacy. It provides appetite control equal to any of the hunger-suppressing medications, with none of their potential drawbacks. It has a salt- and water-eliminating effect that matches the power of diuretic pills without the risk of excess loss of the important mineral potassium, or the rebound retention of salt and water between doses. Fat-burning calms the brain and contributes to the restful sleep that is necessary for energetic days to follow. Finally, ketones, the last of the breakdown products of fat, are in part excreted in the urine, where they can be detected with a product called Ketostix, manufactured by the Ames Company. More on that later—but for now, if you test positive for ketones on arising and at bedtime, you will know that your insulin status has been satisfactory that day, allowing you to burn significant amounts of fat.

CALORIE VERSUS CARBOHYDRATE COUNTING

The body needs energy to maintain its many functions. Its two major fuels are carbohydrate and fat. Because little energy can be stored as carbohydrate, further surplus energy must be held in reserve as fat. It is this energy, stored as fat, that we will be releasing through ketosis.

Calorie (kilocalorie) is the unit used to express a quantity of energy. Carbohydrate and protein provide 4 calories per gram. Protein is rarely used as fuel except in extreme starvation. Fat is more calorie-dense, providing 9 calories per gram. The aim of healthy weight loss is to reduce body fat with minimal loss of precious protein. To lose fat requires a deficit of calories. Since 1 pound of fat contains 3,500 calories, it is obvious that someone who burns 2,000 calories a day and eats only 1,000 will lose 2 pounds of fat a week. This will happen whether or not the diet is low in carbohydrates. The reduction in hunger that accompanies a low-carbohydrate intake, however, makes it easier to stay on the program. Carbohydrate intake must be reduced to 40 grams or less to achieve the state of ketosis indicating that insulin has been reduced enough to liberate fat from storage. Details of the desirable low-carbohydrate diet are contained in chapter 10, "How to Succeed Immediately." Besides control of carbohydrates, fat calories must also be restricted. A low-carbohydrate, ketogenic program that puts no limits on fats needlessly delays reduction of stored body fat. Low-carbohydrate diets are frequently and erroneously described as "high protein." In fact, the amount of protein scarcely exceeds that consumed in a normal diet designed to maintain weight. Only by comparison with the reduced carbohydrate and fat content of the weight-loss diet does that protein seem excessive. This dietary protein is essential, as it cannot be provided by internal sources. Restricting carbohydrate takes priority over the other elements of the diet, but adequate protein and limited intake of fats are also important. Knowing your insulin status through daily ketone testing will help you stay on track.

PUTTING KETOSIS INTO PRACTICE

Seriously overweight people have lost control of their bodies' natural balance. Excessive insulin produced by the pancreas, in response to improper metabolism of sugars, has led to sodium and water retention and inability to utilize the body's stored fat. Within a short period of time, the Insulin Control Diet returns the body to a normal balance. Insulin production is greatly reduced, and the body begins to break down its fat deposits and use that fat for energy. After an initial week or two of dramatic—largely water weight— loss, women can expect to lose 2 to 3 pounds each week and men 3 to 4 pounds weekly. The rate of loss will depend on the amount of excess weight, your age, the amount you exercise, and other individual differences. The most significant aspect of your success with the Insulin Control Diet is that you will lose mostly fat.

Only muscle tissue has a significant capacity to burn calories, thus using food for energy. Fat, on the other hand, is food and can only provide, rather than consume, calories. Men normally need to eat more calories than women because they have a larger metabolic "engine"—namely, larger muscle mass. You want to keep all the lean muscle you can in order to burn more calories during and after your weight loss.

Muscle gives us shape. As we replace fat tissue with lean tissue, not only do we lose pounds, but also inches; therefore, you can measure your progress with both a scale and a tape measure. Today, before you start on the program, take measurements of your waist, hips, thighs, chest, and arms and record them in a journal. (The journal is crucial to being able to follow your progress over time; it is also a practical and easy way to motivate yourself.) You will soon be seeing a dramatic difference.

Several well-known diets of the past have resulted in loss of large amounts of weight, but much lean protein tissue was lost at the same time. This muscle loss was not restricted to the arms and legs. Heart muscle was lost as well, which led to irregular rhythms of the heart—sometimes, even fatally. Since then, protein-sparing diets, which achieve rapid weight loss without significant loss of muscle, have been developed and found to be safe and satisfactory. With the addition of carbohydrate restriction, the Insulin Control Diet has brought these medically proven methods employing low-calorie, protein-supplemented diets to a higher level of patient satisfaction. The most notable advantage is that after no more than three days of adhering to the program, you will experience *almost no hunger whatsoever.*

The diet prescription contains from 800 to 1,200 calories daily, yet you will not be hungry. During the first three days (or less) of following the Insulin Control Diet, the amount of insulin your body produces will drop dramatically, while the amount of glucagon will increase substantially. The body will produce ketones, which curb feelings of hunger. In the place of glucose—blood sugar—your body will also use those ketones as brain fuel. A great benefit of this program is that you will be able to conveniently and inexpensively monitor your body's adaptation by measuring ketones in your urine on a regular basis with the use of Ketostix, which test for the presence of ketones in your urine; you will have visible proof that the diet is working.

On the Insulin Control Diet, what you *do not* eat is far more important than what you *do* eat. While complex carbohydrates are certainly healthful in the form of breads, cereals, fruits, and vegetables, the overweight person's body cannot discriminate between complex and simple sugars. Therefore, simple sugars—such as table sugar—and complex carbohydrates—such as pastas, cereals, and fruits—both will result in the same insidious cycle of insulin release, sodium and fluid retention, fat storage, weight gain, and discouragement. For a brief time, it is necessary to restrict severely the amount of all carbohydrates entering the body.

During the weight-loss period, you will be eating substantial quantities of protein-rich foods, including meats, fish, and poultry. These foods provide nourishment without carbohydrates. They also provide a defense against the excessive protein loss from muscle tissue that is normally seen in rapid weight loss, especially during fasting.

A WORD OF CAUTION

Because protracted mild ketosis in pregnancy may be harmful to the developing fetus, a ketogenic diet should be discontinued once pregnancy is diagnosed. (Temporary ketosis poses no danger to early fetal development, however, and should not be a cause for concern in a woman with polycystic ovarian disorder who is on the Insulin Control Diet to help her get pregnant.)

TESTING FOR KETONES

Testing your urine with Ketostix is a convenient way of verifying that insulin has been reduced sufficiently to liberate large amounts of fat. You can collect urine in a container, dip the plastic stick into the sample, and fifteen seconds later check the color of the stick against a chart on the container. Many people prefer to merely hold the Ketostix in the urine stream to moisten the tip of the strip, as there is no need to soak the strip. The meanings of the various colors are:

- beige: negative ketosis
- pink: mild ketosis
- purple: moderate ketosis
- deeper purple: significant ketosis

On this program, you can expect to see the pink to light purple colors, indicating a state of mild ketosis. You will know when your body begins to free itself from the Metabolic Trap of Obesity as the colors on the Ketostix begin to change. You should test your urine twice daily, preferably once in the morning and once in the evening. You will be able to gauge your progress, and will remain motivated to follow the diet.

On 20 to 35 grams of carbohydrate daily, ketones should appear in two to four days. The falling level of insulin will increase salt and water loss even before ketone positivity appears, and will also reduce appetite, making dieting easier. Weight may drop from 6 to 12 pounds in the first two weeks from the burning of fat, plus the loss of salt and water. Thereafter, weight will fall more slowly because less excess fluid remains to be eliminated.

With carbohydrates and fats restricted in this program, it is easy to assume that salt should also be avoided. This would be a mistake that could lead to serious consequences. There is a significant loss of salt in the urine on a ketogenic diet; unless this is replaced by salty foods or a daily supplement of about 1 teaspoon of table salt, blood pressure will often fall sufficiently to cause faintness on standing and possible injury.

Testing for ketones on arising and at bedtime gives valuable information in addition to the level of insulin in the system. For example, when there is little or no weight loss despite an apparent strict adherence to the program, it is helpful to know if ketones are still present. If they are, it means that fat is being burned as expected, but significant water retention is masking the fat loss. This weight plateau is fairly common in women and is often related to the menstrual cycle. Vigorous exercise, by diverting blood away from the kidneys to muscles, may decrease water excretion and add to the fluid retention. Therefore, it is comforting to know that fat is still being burned and that more exercise at this time is not called for, as it may aggravate the situation.

Tracking your ketones also enables you to safely increase the variety of carbohydrate foods you consume. If you replace one carbohydrate with another and still stay in ketosis, then the switch is satisfactory. If ketones disappear, however, then another choice should be made.

Usually, within three days of entering the program, the Ketostix will turn a light shade of pink or purple, indicating that you have entered a mild state of ketosis. On the Insulin Control Diet, the ketosis remains mild, never developing into a state severe enough to pose potential damage. Ketones in the urine are an indirect measurement of insulin in the blood. Ideally, you should measure them on arising and at bedtime while on the weight-loss program, as previously suggested. If you go out of ketosis, examine your actions to see what you might have done to cause this, and try to correct the situation. Ketostix can also be regarded as your portable conscience that will help you stay on the right path. If you fail to lose weight for a week or two, even though ketones remain positive, you are retaining fluid for some reason or other; this should not be a cause for concern, as it is usually only temporary. This temporary retention of water weight is dealt with in chapter 6, "The Ins and Outs of Salt and Water."

What does it mean when Ketostix, previously showing light purple consistently, suddenly turns dark purple? It indicates that the urine has become concentrated due to water deficiency rather than increased production of ketones. The proper response is to increase fluid intake until the urine is more diluted.

SUMMARY

- Ketosis is a process of fat burning in which your body converts fat calories into energy.
- The burning of fat calories makes for a "beneficial natural pharmacy" while you lose weight.
- The use of Ketostix, manufactured by the Ames Company, will allow you to monitor your body's insulin level and ensure that you are burning fat calories.
- The mild state of ketosis into which the diet will place your body is safe and maintainable.

CHAPTER 5

Desperately Seeking Serotonin

THERE ARE A NUMBER OF NATURAL chemicals that affect food intake. The most important, from a practical standpoint, is the brain-communicating chemical (neurotransmitter) serotonin. Chapter 1 presented serotonin's role in curbing carbohydrate cravings and promoting deep, restorative sleep. Now, I want to expand on the influence and importance of serotonin and how we can modify it to our advantage.

There are three ways of increasing the effectiveness of serotonin: sleep, carbohydrate intake, and the use of prescription medications called SSRIs (selective serotonin reuptake inhibitors). Only the first, sleep, is truly helpful. Deep, restorative sleep requires some serotonin to take place. In normal individuals studied in a sleep lab, normal sleep is best described like going underwater. Shallow or superficial sleep is characterized by much dreaming, with the eyes tracking dreams on a mental screen. This rapid eye movement (REM) sleep is necessary for a portion of the night but is not deep enough to restore the chemical balance of the brain sufficiently for optimum performance the next day. After sleeping only at this level, you will begin the day feeling tired.

You require deeper levels of sleep under the influence of serotonin to replenish all your neurotransmitters with maximum efficiency. At this deep-sleep level, serotonin itself is also enhanced. The way you feel, think, and act the next day is determined by the quality of the previous night's sleep. Normally, you should start the morning energized, and follow it with a cheerful and productive afternoon and evening.

The store of serotonin in the brain is often depleted by chronic stress. Nonrestorative sleep follows, with no natural way of readily replenishing adequate serotonin. A small external source of serotonin at bedtime is needed to jump-start the sleep system. Tryptophan, the amino-acid building block of serotonin, was employed in this role until ten years ago, when it was linked to a worldwide epidemic of a sometimes-fatal neuromuscular disorder. The disease appeared to be due to product contamination in a Japanese factory making much of the world's supply of tryptophan; because of the close similarities of the "good" and "bad" tryptophan, however, the safety of tryptophan and its related counterpart, 5-hydroxytryptophan, have been challenged and they are no longer used freely.

A more satisfactory source of serotonin at bedtime is the old-fashioned antidepressant trazodone. Twenty years ago, when it was often prescribed, the dose for mood elevation ranged from 400 to 600 milligrams. This frequently produced side effects, such as dry mouth, constipation, and a drop in blood pressure on standing to the point of faintness. When the new generation of antidepressants with fewer side effects—led by Prozac—became available, trazodone was abandoned as a treatment for depression. In our clinic, we use a small dose (25 to 50 milligrams) to provide sufficient serotonin to begin the process of deep, restorative sleep. Imagine serotonin as being stored in a brain reservoir, which because of chronic stress is nearly empty; the challenge is to begin to fill it.

A good night's sleep adds to the level of serotonin in the reservoir. This process continues with each night's sleep until after a time—often several months—enough is available internally so that little or no external supplementation is needed. All the while, serotonin levels remain sufficient to control carbohydrate cravings, which in turn allows insulin to remain reduced.

Carbohydrate feeding is another way to increase your serotonin temporarily. How does this happen? The brain is covered by a "curtain" that separates it from the main bloodstream. It is called the blood/brain barrier, and it is penetrated by a limited number of small openings that regulate which substances can enter and leave the brain. Amino acids, which are derived from protein, are the building blocks of the neurotransmitters; there are twenty-two amino acids in humans. They are in competition with each other for the privilege of entering the brain through the limited number of openings in the blood/brain barrier. Insulin is not only the blood sugar–lowering hormone; it also lowers the blood level of amino acids, with one important exception—tryptophan. Carbohydrate feeding increases insulin, which temporarily eliminates the other twenty-one amino acids. This removal of competition allows tryptophan to enter the brain freely to produce a rapid, but short-lived, increase in serotonin. The effect of this burst of serotonin can vary from calmness and comfort to extreme drowsiness, particularly if serotonin has been quite deficient prior to the carbohydrate ingestion. The rise in serotonin is only temporary and adds nothing to the depleted reservoir— what does remain are the added calories that have been ingested.

There is a common misconception that hypoglycemia (an abnormal lack of blood sugar) is a frequent cause of mental disturbance that is relieved by eating carbohydrate. True hypoglycemia (which can be verified by checking the blood sugar) occurs fairly frequently in insulin-treated diabetics or those on oral medication that can lower the blood sugar by acting like insulin. An exceedingly rare cause is an insulin-producing tumor. Many patients diagnose themselves as hypoglycemic because their nervous symptoms are relieved by ingesting carbohydrate.

There is no doubt that carbohydrate makes them feel better, but it is likely that increased serotonin, by providing a natural tranquilizing effect, deserves the credit for the improvement.

Sometimes SSRIs, such as Prozac, are recommended for serotonin enhancement in weight-loss programs. The results have been disappointing. The mode of action of these drugs is to prevent the inactivation of serotonin that normally occurs after one passage across the gap (synapse) that separates two nerve cells. Inactivation requires serotonin be taken up by the nerve cell from which it originated. Inhibiting the reuptake allows serotonin to traverse the synapse more than once, adding to its effect; however, there is no increase in the amount of serotonin and no addition is made to the serotonin reservoir.

Because many obese patients are depressed, SSRIs also have been used to elevate mood; they only recycle existing serotonin levels, however, and should not be counted on to improve the quality of sleep or to curb carbohydrate cravings. In these cases, bedtime trazodone should be used, sometimes in conjunction with a daytime SSRI. There is no harm in the combination, as long as the doses employed are carefully monitored, recognizing that each tends to somewhat alter the other's effect. SSRIs can also inhibit sleep patterns, as they have a stimulating effect. I tell my patients who are taking SSRIs that if they're having difficulty sleeping, they should not take the medication after noon; preferably they should take it as early in the morning as possible in order for the medication to have the least effect on their sleep.

SEROTONIN EXCESS

Even though serotonin deficiency can be troublesome, it does not directly produce structural changes in the body—not so with serotonin excess. In rare cases of serotonin-producing tumors, damage to the heart valves has been observed. Similar but milder changes occurred in many patients treated with the appetite-suppressing drugs fenfluramine and dexfenfluramine, which act by increasing the release of stored serotonin. Because of these changes, the FDA ordered their withdrawal. Still authorized for appetite control is phentermine, the remaining partner of the phen-fen combination. It is a member of the amphetamine family, whose actions include central nervous system stimulation and elevation of blood pressure.

Sibutramine, another drug recently introduced for management of obesity, produces its effects by inhibiting the reuptake of serotonin, noradrenaline, and dopamine. Although there have been no cases of valvular heart disease associated with extended use, this drug substantially increases blood pressure in some patients; therefore, blood pressure should be regularly monitored. Sibutramine does control appetite, but it does not add to the serotonin reservoir any more than the less effective antidepressant SSRIs. As mentioned previously, in the long run, the most effective serotonin replenisher seems to be low-dose trazodone, working through creation of a good night's sleep.

When you decide to begin the Insulin Control Diet, your physician must be a participant, as you'll need a prescription for trazodone. In addition, it will be helpful for a medical professional to be overseeing your progress on the program. However, you can be your own weight-loss doctor for most of the practical decisions that this course of treatment requires (see chapter 8).

SUMMARY

- Deep, restorative sleep is necessary for the replenishment of your serotonin supply.
- You must rebuild your body's supply of serotonin in order to overcome carbohydrate cravings. When your serotonin has

been restored, you will be on the path to permanent weight loss.

- A small dose of trazodone is recommended to achieve deep sleep and the replenishment of serotonin. Consult with your physician for prescriptions and the supervision of a medical professional.

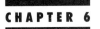

CHAPTER 6

The Ins and Outs of Salt and Water

NORMAL BLOOD AND TISSUE LEVELS OF SALT (sodium) and water are needed for good health. We continuously lose water and salt in a variety of ways, however. The biggest loss is through excretion in the urine, which is regulated by hormones. With regard to salt, the excessive insulin that is characteristic of obesity is a powerful influence for retaining salt and accompanying water. When this effect is drastically reduced by the Insulin Control Diet, considerable salt and water are excreted, producing an often dramatic weight loss. The accompanying decrease in circulating blood volume, however, which is normally required to maintain blood pressure (particularly on standing up), may produce light-headedness and a tendency to faint when arising suddenly. For this reason, salt should *not* be restricted on the Insulin Control Diet. In fact, *at least 1 teaspoon of table salt or its equivalent in salty foods should be ingested daily.* Many patients with hypertension are still taking diuretics, usually as part of their treatment (sometimes with additional potassium to replace excessive losses). In these cases, the dose of diuretic should probably be reduced; if the blood pressure remains normal, the drug may be withdrawn.

Weight loss may be interrupted by a plateau of fluid retention, particularly in women. The most obvious causes of water-weight gain are premenstrual syndrome, excessive carbohydrate intake, and inappropriate secretion of the water-retaining pituitary hormone (vasopressin or antidiuretic hormone, ADH, which reduces the kidney's ability to excrete water). If there is no weight loss but the urine remains positive for ketones, it means you are burning fat as expected but replacing it with equivalent weight in water. If you are no longer in ketosis, then carbohydrate has somehow crept into your diet, or there has been a sufficient secretion of insulin-antagonizing stress hormones to require more insulin for blood-sugar control. This extra insulin then takes you out of ketosis and causes you to retain salt and water.

As mentioned, stress can make you gain water weight another way—through increased secretion of vasopressin. The hypothalamus, a portion of the brain that lies above and controls the pituitary gland, contains several regulatory centers. Two that exert the most influential control of the ins and outs of water are the osmostat and the thirst center. The osmostat is a group of nerve cells sensitive to minor changes in the osmotic pressure (or concentration) of the blood, which is determined mainly by its water content and the amount of electrolytes (chiefly sodium) that it carries. An increase in osmotic pressure triggers the release of vasopressin, which then causes water retention. The nerve cells that make vasopressin are located in the hypothalamus but terminate in the neural portion of the pituitary gland, where the hormone is stored for immediate release, if necessary, to act on the kidney and retain water. The thirst center is less sensitive than the osmostat to fluid concentration, but it does help to replenish fluid deficits by stimulating drinking.

Finally, excessive exercise can also cause water retention, especially in women. It does so by shunting blood away from the kidneys to the muscles, thereby decreasing the kidneys' ability to excrete fluids. The bottom line is that if you are still in ketosis, don't always rely on the scale, as it cannot differentiate between fat and water.

DIABETES INSIPIDUS

In the uncommon disease diabetes insipidus (water diabetes), which may result from brain injury or a tumor in the hypothalamic area or pituitary gland, there is a deficient manufacture, or release, of vasopressin. Excessive urination (polyuria) and increased thirst (polydipsia) are the cardinal features of the disease. A much rarer form of this disorder, nephrogenic (meaning "from the kidney") diabetes insipidus, which is sometimes familial, results from a defect in the cells of the kidney tubules that normally reabsorb water under the influence of vasopressin. Other more common and less severe forms of nephrogenic diabetes insipidus are caused by drugs (e.g., lithium and the antibiotic demeclocycline), which can block the action of vasopressin, as can increased levels of calcium. Measuring the blood level of vasopressin by radioimmunoassay distinguishes between central (hypothalamic/pituitary) diabetes insipidus and the nephrogenic form. In the latter form, the vasopressin level is elevated, in contrast to its near absence in the central form. The other test of value in managing these conditions is the serum osmolality, which can often be approximated by multiplying serum sodium by 2 and adding 10. In diabetes insipidus of any origin, the sodium and osmolality are usually elevated.

Sometimes, excessive thirst (polydipsia) of emotional origin, or due to a chronically dry mouth from inadequate salivary secretion, can mimic diabetes insipidus. In this case, however, the polyuria is secondary to the primary polydipsia. In these patients, drinking is usually somewhat ahead of urination and therefore the blood is often somewhat dilute, but never is the osmolality increased above normal.

DIURETIC DRUGS

Diuretic drugs are well known to increase excretion of salt, taking water with it. Most diuretics also eliminate some potassium, while a few are reputed to be potassium sparing. The most powerful salt-retaining agent of the body, even more so than insulin, is the adrenal hormone aldosterone. While aldosterone causes sodium retention, it also causes significant amounts of potassium to be excreted. The chief stimulus to aldosterone excretion is a decreasing circulating-blood volume, which is the usual effect of diuretics, even those that are supposed to spare potassium. Therefore, chronic diuretic use should include supplemental potassium and appropriate determinations of serum potassium to see if replenishment is adequate. Sufficiently low potassium can result in electrical instability of the heart, with the danger of fatal cardiac arrest.

WATER INTOXICATION

Fluid retention is not confined to your extremities and abdomen. It also affects your brain, interfering subtly with its functions. It can be said that fluid retention "clouds the mind," producing water intoxication.

DIURESIS OF RECUMBENCY

To increase loss of salt and water weight during the period of ketosis, I recommend the simple measure of achieving diuresis through recumbency; that is, excreting water from the tissues by urinating, a process that can be enhanced by merely resting propped up at a 45-degree angle (recumbent) for between thirty minutes and two hours each day. It is best to do this in the middle of the day, when your body is most susceptible to the technique. After resting for at least thirty minutes, you should arise feeling relaxed and that you need to urinate.

Because water weight is already being shed through ketosis, diuresis of recumbency is an optional technique; however, it can be helpful in dealing with "plateaus" of fluid retention that are not responding well to ketosis. By expelling water weight through this method, you will be able to immediately shed as much as a pound of water.

SUMMARY

- Don't be discouraged if you don't initially lose weight, even when your Ketostix indicate that you are in ketosis. If you are in a state of ketosis, you *are* burning fat weight; most likely the retention of water is keeping your weight constant. Retention of water weight is temporary.
- In order to shed water weight, try diuresis of recumbency. You should immediately be able to shed up to a pound of water weight.
- At least 1 teaspoon of table salt or its equivalent in salty foods should be ingested daily while on the Insulin Control Diet in order to maintain normal tissue levels of sodium.

CHAPTER 7

Diabesity: The Link Between Obesity and Diabetes

THERE ARE AT LEAST 16 MILLION DIABETICS in the United States. Less than 10 percent depend on insulin for their survival, and they are classified as Type 1. The others produce considerable internal insulin, but are resistant to it. Ninety percent of these Type 2 diabetics are significantly overweight; that is, more than 20 percent above ideal body weight. We believe there are an equal number of Type 2 diabetics not yet diagnosed, who are still exposed to the progressive deterioration that gradually produces complications of diabetes. In the United States, diabetes is now the leading cause of blindness, kidney failure, and amputations for threatened or established gangrene.

The total cost of health care for the nation's diabetics has been estimated to be over $50 billion annually. Add to that the cost of diminished productivity from lost time from work, estimated to be another $25 billion, and you can see that caring for diabetics consumes a very large part of our national wealth.

Type 2 diabetes and obesity are closely linked. To alert and alarm them, I tell my overweight patients that they are "not yet diabetics." Some of them, because of a strong family history of obesity-related Type 2 diabetes, already know this. But heredity need not become destiny if insulin resistance can be contained.

Type 2 diabetics predominantly are insulin resistant, but they also have a diminished capacity to produce extra insulin when needed. The pancreas, which essentially acts as an "insulin factory," becomes less efficient with aging. When the pancreas can no longer meet the demand for additional insulin, the blood sugar rises significantly, making the diagnosis of diabetes very obvious.

Type 2 diabetics have a form of insulin resistance that is independent of obesity. We know this because a small number of normal-weight patients have this disease. The cause of this inherited resistance is still unknown, but it is under intensive investigation. Obesity is another powerful source of insulin resistance. If a significant amount of weight is gained, for whatever reason—stopping smoking, depression, decreased activity, or steroid treatment for an inflammatory or allergic condition—fat then produces more TNF-alpha. Thus, fat begets more fat. If sufficient weight is gained, and if aging reduces the pancreas's ability to produce sufficient amounts of insulin, then diabetes will result. There are at least three times as many significantly obese people as there are diabetics in the United States. Most of these individuals can be considered "prediabetic."

What can be done to reduce the mounting cases of both obesity and diabetes, which, alarmingly, are affecting more and more children and adolescents? *Weight loss!* Weight loss is always prescribed for obese patients, but it is rarely achieved because insulin control is not aggressively applied. If the Insulin Control Diet were widely employed, impressive inroads could be made in prevention and management of obesity and its major complication, Type 2 diabetes. Sufficient weight loss has reversed diabetes in many of our obese patients. What follows are excerpts from an interview with Judd, a patient who came to me overweight and diagnosed with Type 2 diabetes. Prior treatment for the condition was failing, and his diabetes had already been determined to require additional medication for its control

Judd: I've always liked to eat, okay? Up until the time I was about twenty-five or twenty-eight, I bounced between 165 and 175. I had taken up weightlifting. I used to swim tremendous amounts. I used to play clarinet and saxophone semiprofessionally. I grew up and was educated in Chicago. You know, when you're young and still basically in shape, you don't have a weight problem. But as I got older and my metabolism slowed down, I began putting on weight. And then, in about the early 1980s, I was up around 185 to 190, and I'm a little guy. I'm only about 5' 5½", and I wasn't working out. I was working a high-stress job—life insurance agent, financial planner—and have been for about thirty-two years. Folks, it's kind of stressful with all the changes in the communities: the financial community, the planning community. I just got heavier and heavier. If I had a good day, when I would come home, after dinner, I would celebrate via food. If I had a bad day, I would console myself with food. I was of that generation of people where the grandmas and grandpas always said, "Eat, eat."

About 1985, I had gotten up to around 205, 210, and I've always been blessed with tremendous amounts of energy, even now. Then about the middle of 1988, I noticed really significant levels of being tired, just being tired. I had never been tired in my life. At that time, I was about 215. Surprisingly, as a life insurance guy quite familiar with many medical conditions, I never thought of diabetes. Then, a remarkable thing happened in the early part of 1989—I started losing weight. I'd never lost weight before. So I went and saw my GP, and my triglycerides were about 700 to 750, total cholesterol was close to 300, blood sugar was around 185. He says, "Congratulations, you've got diabetes! You're Type 2, you've got to lose some weight." He gave me some oral medication, and I felt great for about two months. Then, the symptoms started returning.

I came up here, to see Dr. Ezrin. At the end of about a fifteen-minute meeting, he explained to me what he thought I had, which was strange since there were no blood tests, no workup, nothing. He says, "It looks like you're insulin resistant, grossly obese." Then he made a statement which was clear. I understand the English language quite well. He said, "Untreated diabetes is eventually terminal." I heard that.

Judd went on the Insulin Control Diet shortly before the end of 1989; by April 1990, he was down to 162 pounds. His blood sugar had entered a normal range and his insulin level was even lower than normal; the symptoms of diabetes were gone. He no longer takes any medication, and exercises daily by riding a stationary bike: "Like breathing, I do that every day."

Judd: I did a complete lifestyle change. I realized that although diabetes was an unwelcome partner, and one that I wanted to get rid of, it was my companion. And now I feel, now I know, that Type 2 diabetes was a blessing in disguise because I'm sure I would have had a heart attack, or worse, if I hadn't changed my lifestyle. I'm sure of it.

In patients with diabesity, the first-line treatment is weight loss, which will render further drug therapy unnecessary in many cases; however, good control of diabetes, proven by a consistently satisfactory hemoglobin A1C (a measure of the average blood sugar for the preceding three months), is still the most important goal. If possible, this should be achieved with the least amount of insulin—either internal or external. In those instances where insulin is required to achieve satisfactory control of blood sugar, it should not be withheld too long lest the persistent hyperglycemia (high blood sugar) add further to the risk of diabetic complications.

An increased frequency of cardiovascular disease appears to be one of the major consequences of insulin resistance and hyperinsulinemia. This is even more pronounced in patients with Type 2 diabetes. Cardiovascular disease includes hypertension and atherosclerosis, or arteriosclerosis involving the coronary arteries and the cerebral vessels. Abnormalities of fat metabolism are important cardiovascular risk factors. Elevated cholesterol and low-density lipoproteins (LDL) are associated with an increased incidence of coronary heart disease, while high-density lipoproteins (HDL) seem to protect the heart against the ravages of bad cholesterol. Triglyclerides and very low density lipoproteins (VLDL) also appear to independently contribute to coronary heart disease. Insulin is closely associated with triglycerides and HDL, as it raises blood levels of triglycerides and decreases HDL manufactured by the liver.

The trio of hyperinsulinemia, raised triglycerides and LDL levels, and decreased HDL cholesterol levels is a common finding in patients with cardiovascular disease. Hypertension is an additional risk factor. When diabetes is added to the mix, the risk of stroke or heart attack with resultant serious disability and even a fatal outcome is increased enormously.

Ten years ago, Robert Kowalski (an esteemed science writer and author of the bestselling *8-Week Cholesterol Cure*) and I collaborated on our first book dealing with the role of insulin resistance in obesity. When we landed in my hometown, Toronto, Canada, at the end of a national book-promoting tour, we were interviewed by Wilder Penfield III, a well-known columnist for the *Globe and Mail.* In his report the next day of the encounter, Penfield wrote that our collaboration was a marriage made in diet heaven. I enjoyed the hyperbole and promised to remember it forever. I recall that incident because I wanted to end this chapter with something equally memorable: I believe that the relationship between obesity and diabetes is like a marriage made in diet hell, and the divorce rate is alarmingly low.

CHAPTER 8

How to Be Your Own Weight-Loss Doctor

IN THE MEDICAL TREATMENT OF OBESITY, the patient is much more important than the doctor. Success depends more on the patient's understanding and cooperation than any medication prescribed. Physicians can serve their significantly overweight patients best by convincing them to take effective action and keeping them out of harm's way while they are reducing. How can an overweight layperson best help herself to become lightened? By becoming enlightened!

Food calories come largely from fat and carbohydrate. The body needs only a very small amount of food fat—just enough to supply essential fatty acids that the body cannot produce. No carbohydrate is essential in the diet, if vitamins, minerals, and fiber are supplied as supplements. At least 7 to 10 ounces of protein must be eaten daily, because the body cannot make protein from internal sources alone. Based on these dietary needs, the composition of your reducing diet will be mainly protein, with very little fat or carbohydrate. High-protein diets are sometimes said to be damaging to the kidneys, but there is no more protein in the Insulin Control Diet than in an ordinary diet. Furthermore, protein is not dangerous for normal kidneys.

The Insulin Control Diet contains fewer calories than your body spends; apart from the few calories that come from an initial small amount of carbohydrate, stored fat is the only significant source of energy.

When fat is the body's major source of energy, weight loss becomes easier because of better appetite control. If you test your ketones regularly, you will always know if insulin is being reduced sufficiently to produce maximum benefit. I regard urine ketone testing in this program as important in providing useful medical information as home blood glucose monitoring is for diabetics striving for optimal blood sugar control.

Carbohydrate restriction is more important than calorie reduction, although the ultimate rate of fat loss depends on a negative balance of calories. The meal plans listed in this book provide 800 to 1,200 calories daily, with carbohydrate restricted to less than 40 grams. On a 1,000-calorie diet, when the body requires 2,500 calories to support its energy needs, 1,500 calories will be provided from fat stores. In a sense, you will be consuming your own fat, in a manner equivalent to intravenous fat feeding. Therefore, if you are challenged about the safety and sufficiency of your diet, you can respond that you are really being fed 2,500 calories—1,000 by mouth and 1,500 from your own fat. The internal fat feeding is much healthier than the equivalent of animal fat that would be eaten. In addition to the beneficial natural pharmacy that it supplies, burning body fat lowers harmful cholesterol. By following the plan described in this book, beginning with the Insulin Control Diet, your fat can be changed from an enemy to a friend.

MEAL PLANS FOR THE WEIGHT-LOSS PHASE

Using the food lists provided in chapter 10, you can compose daily meal plans that are interesting, satisfying, and sufficiently varied to satisfy your needs. In general, women are permitted a daily total of 7 ounces of protein, such as fish, poultry, or lean meat, in addition to one egg or 2 ounces of low-fat cottage cheese; men are permitted 10 ounces. You may also have 2 cups of any nonstarchy vegetable plus one serving of fruit—or, if you prefer, one serving of juice.

On some days, you might substitute one slice of bread or 2 cups of cereal (without milk) for your serving of fruit. You may partake of a wide variety of greens, such as lettuce and spinach, and use other free vegetables (e.g., radishes, mushrooms, and green onions) to provide color and added enjoyment to your two daily salads.

Because of their lactose (milk sugar) content, both milk and yogurt, the chief sources of calcium in the diet, are completely eliminated during the weight-loss phase of the Insulin Control Diet. To provide the calcium needed to maintain bone health, a *daily supplement of 1,000 milligrams (1 gram) of calcium is required.*

The weight-loss phase of the diet contains no added fat or oil. Eat only lean meats and trim all visible fat from each serving. Use cooking methods that call for little added oil. Food should be baked, broiled, steamed, poached, or boiled, rather than fried or sautéed.

To obtain all the vitamins, minerals, and trace nutrients your body requires while you are limiting food intake, you will need a daily vitamin and mineral supplement. Because you will be eliminating large amounts of water and sodium, salt should be added to the diet to prevent the sodium depletion that can produce light-headedness and faintness on standing. Use a total of 1 teaspoon (5 grams) of salt in cooking or as seasoning.

At first glance, a carbohydrate- and calorie-restricted diet may seem inadequate. When care is taken to provide necessary supplements, however, nothing significant will be lacking in your diet.

Before you embark on a major weight-loss program, your physician should be consulted. Most of the responsibility for success will lie with you, but it will be reassuring to have your doctor overseeing your progress. There are five items that might require your physician's attention:

1. Trazodone for nighttime serotonin enhancement.
2. Adjustment of salt intake if you are on blood pressure medication, particularly if you are taking a diuretic. With weight loss, blood pressure medication can often be reduced.
3. Gallstones are often present in overweight individuals. The gallbladder's normal response to food fat is to contract in order to deliver bile to the intestine, where it aids in fat digestion. In a low-calorie, low-carbohydrate, very fat restricted diet such as Opti-Fast, fat is not available in the diet to stimulate the gallbladder to contract. If the diet is broken with a high-fat meal, however, a sudden violent contraction of the gallbladder can result, dislodging gallstones into the bile duct. This can produce severe pain and can sometimes lead to acute inflammation of the gallbladder. Fortunately, in our program there is enough fat in the protein foods that are the mainstay of the diet to repeatedly stimulate the gallbladder, and there is no significant threat of suddenly discharging silent stones. Still, the danger to the gallbladder posed by a sudden high-fat meal should be remembered as an additional reason to stick to the diet.
4. Uric acid is derived from the breakdown of tissue, including fat. During rapid weight loss, uric acid levels may increase. If they are sufficiently elevated, acute gouty arthritis may

result from deposition of uric acid crystals in the joints. Kidney stones containing uric acid can also form. These adverse events are rare and are more likely to occur in men whose uric acid levels are already high before the weight-loss program is started. Women rarely have gout or significantly elevated uric acid levels; however, it is prudent to consult with your physician and enlist his or her cooperation, including providing a chemistry panel that includes uric acid. Your doctor may wish to prescribe a well-tolerated medication, 150 to 300 milligrams of Allopurinol, to lower elevated uric acid levels.

5. Because of their low carbohydrate intake, diabetics who embark on the Insulin Control Diet will often reduce blood sugar substantially even before much weight has been lost. Further decrease in blood sugar levels occurs with progressive weight loss. Your physician will reduce diabetes medications to adjust for this improvement.

Obviously, anyone seriously interested in an effective, permanent weight-loss program should have a sympathetic physician as a coach, but good, lasting results depend on an engaged, informed subject. To establish an effective doctor/patient relationship, you may first have to convince your physician that what you are proposing has merit and is worth trying. This book was written to help patients and their physicians understand the forces behind the increasing epidemic of obesity. It also describes a very effective low-risk model for managing this disorder. In our hands, this treatment has been very successful, particularly in previously resistant cases. If it were more widely adopted, the trend of increasing weight gain could be readily reversed. Therefore, encourage your doctor to read the explanatory sections of this book.

PART II

CLIMB ABOARD THE KETOSIS EXPRESS

CHAPTER 9

Just the Facts: Your Guide to Basic Nutrition

It seems at every turn, there is more information about nutrition. There are countless publications that trumpet the "miracle" effects of different foods and vitamins. It is often difficult to discern what is fact and what is fiction. This much is true: The foods we choose to put into our bodies do affect our ability to maintain good health. Nutrients are used by the body to repair, build, and maintain body tissue; thus, the old adage "You are what you eat" does contain much truth.

Following is a breakdown of macronutrients (carbohydrate, protein, and fat) and micronutrients (vitamins and minerals) necessary for nutritional balance.

WATER

Water may be the most important nutrient. One-third to one-half of the body's weight is water; without it, we can't survive. Water is essential for maintaining proper hydration and digestion. It is also vital for maintaining electrolyte balance, which in turn is critical to the body's ability to function properly. We lose water through various methods. Urination rids the body of waste material, while perspiration—the body's natural mechanism to regulate temperature—is another way in which the body excretes fluid. Therefore, it is necessary for you to consume fluids throughout the day. A standard recommendation is *eight 8-ounce glasses of water daily.*

As mentioned earlier, insulin is a powerful salt- and water-retaining hormone, so when the body lowers insulin output and enters a state of ketosis, it rids itself of copious amounts of fluid. Although this provides a nice natural diuretic effect, it is necessary to replenish the lost fluids in the body. Drink up!

CARBOHYDRATE

Carbohydrates can be placed into two major categories: simple sugars and complex carbohydrates (starches). Whether you eat a baked potato or a candy bar, the body will break down those foods and convert them to sugar in the blood—namely, glucose. Because of this, carbohydrates, both simple and complex, are restricted during the weight-loss phase of the Insulin Control Diet. But don't be discouraged: during stabilization and maintenance, carbohydrates will be reintroduced into the diet. We advocate choosing complex carbohydrates over simple sugars. In fact, we encourage you to think of simple sugars as poison. Sugars stimulate insulin and elevate the body's production of triglycerides, increasing one's risk for heart disease. Doesn't seem worth it, does it?

Complex carbohydrates provide the body with both insoluble and soluble fiber. Insoluble fiber is that which does not break down into sugars, but rather improves the passage of foods through the gut. Insoluble fiber is found in foods such as wheat, fruit, and vegetables. Soluble fiber has been shown to reduce levels of cholesterol by "attaching" to certain by-products of cholesterol, namely bile acids, and eliminating them from the body. Soluble fiber is found in foods such as oat bran, cornmeal, and dried beans.

FAT

Although it may be hard to believe, fat is a critical component of overall nutritional health; it's necessary to the transportation of fat-soluble vitamins (A, D, E, and K) and it provides the body with energy. Fat cushions vital organs and provides insulation, and it's also involved in the metabolism of food. There is no question that we need fat in the diet; the question is, How much?

Both the American Heart Association and the American Dietetic Association have recommended that fat calories not exceed 30 percent of one's total caloric intake; however, the Western diet derives over 40 percent of its calories from fat! We can have "too much of a good thing." It is important to recognize the types of fats found in the diet, and the role they play in your overall health.

Fats can be classified as saturated, polyunsaturated, and mono-unsaturated. High concentrations of saturated fats are found in animal products such as butter and lard (or products that include these); beef, pork, and lamb; and coconut and palm oils. Saturated fats have been associated with atherosclerosis (hardening of the arteries) and increased risk of cancer. It is recommended that no more than 10 percent of fat calories come from saturated fats.

Polyunsaturated fats, found in vegetable oils, have been shown to be somewhat neutral. Monounsaturated fats found in olive and canola oil are also neutral. In other words, these fats cause no major changes to cholesterol levels. Your fats of choice should be polyunsaturated fat and monounsaturated fat.

VITAMINS AND MINERALS

Vitamins and minerals are critical nutrients that are involved in all body processes. Most people are familiar with the recommended dietary allowance (RDA) for vitamins and minerals; but what do the recommendations mean? For the average person, RDAs are based on the amounts of vitamins and minerals needed to prevent deficiencies that could lead to serious health complications. In theory, if one consumes a healthy, balanced diet, supplementation may not be necessary; however, the Western diet is rarely "balanced" or—for that matter—"healthy." It is highly unlikely that you get all the nutrients you need at a fast-food restaurant. Because certain food groups are restricted during the weight-loss phase of the Insulin Control Diet, supplementation is highly recommended.

There are thirteen vitamins that occur naturally in food. Of these, four are fat-soluble and are stored in fat tissue: A, D, E, and K. The remaining nine vitamins are water-soluble. If the body receives copious amounts of water-soluble vitamins, it will simply excrete unneeded amounts in the urine.

There are fifteen minerals essential in your diet. RDAs have been established for six of these minerals: calcium, phosphorus, iodine, iron, magnesium, and zinc. The remaining minerals are needed in lesser amounts. In this chapter, the roles of copper and chromium in your diet will also be discussed. Table 9.1 gives a brief overview of the functions of certain vitamins and minerals. Tables 9.2 through 9.4 give daily dietary allowances and show how much of the major nutrients you should consume.

Table 9.1 Vitamins and Minerals

Vitamin/Mineral	Source	Function
Vitamin A	Vegetables, including carrots and sweet potatoes	Involved in body cell-building processes and necessary for the prevention of certain eye diseases
Vitamin D	Dairy products and fish	Aids in building bone tissue and in absorbing calcium in the digestive tract
Vitamin E	Vegetable oils, butterfat, egg yolks, green leafy vegetables, whole grains, wheat germ	Functions as an antioxidant in the cells and tissues of the body
Vitamin K	Spinach, cabbage, and liver	Essential in blood clotting, and is produced by intestinal flora (bacteria in the gastrointestinal tract)
Vitamin C	Fruits and vegetables	Increases the body's healing process and improves its resistance to infection; involved in the formation and repair of collagen, a connective tissue that holds tissues and cells together
Vitamin B_1 (thiamine)	Nuts, whole-grain foods, pork	Contributes to immune system and nervous system functions
Vitamin B_2 (riboflavin)	Milk, yogurt, cottage cheese	Promotes healthy eyes and skin; works in concert with other B vitamins in the metabolism of carbo-hydrates, proteins, and fats
Vitamin B_3 (niacin or nicotinamide)	Yeast, peanuts, meats, fish, poultry, whole-grain products	Involved in the metabolism of foods

Continued overleaf

Table 9.1 Vitamins and Minerals, *continued*

Vitamin/Mineral	Source	Function
Vitamin B_6 (pyridoxine)	Soybeans, lima beans, bananas, whole-grain cereals, various meats	Promotes the metabolism of proteins and its component substances; namely, amino acids; pyridoxine is also involved in the manufacture of compounds such as hormones, hemoglobin, and antibodies
Vitamin B_{12} (cyanocobalamin)	Found only in animal products such as fish, meat, and dairy products	Necessary for blood formation and is involved in the maintenance of nervous tissue; B_{12} is absorbed in the gut with the help of a substance known as intrinsic factor; without this substance, individuals lack B_{12} and may develop pernicious anemia
Folic acid (folacin or folate)	Green leafy vegetables, nuts, legumes	Assists in maintaining nervous tissue and blood cells; pregnant women require more folate during pregnancy to prevent neural tube defects such as spina bifida
Biotin	Milk, liver, legumes, egg yolk, yeast	Involved in carbohydrate metabolism
Pantothenic acid	Eggs, salmon, organ meats, wheat bran, yeast, peanuts; vegetables are also a good source of pantothenic acid	Involved in food metabolism

Calcium	Found most abundantly in dairy products; other sources include sardines, some shellfish, and green leafy vegetables	Ensures bone health and is required for regulatory functions in the blood serum; supplementation of calcium can reduce the odds of developing osteoporosis (a bone-demineralizing disease); we recommend 1,000 mg calcium daily, although needs may be higher for women who are menopausal or postmenopausal and on hormone replacement
Iron	Beef and fortified cereals	When combined with protein, forms hemoglobin that transports oxygen throughout the body; needs may be greater during menstruation; vitamin C supplementation improves the absorption of iron
Phosphorus	Milk, fish, eggs, poultry, meat, legumes; soft drinks are also a source of phosphorus	High amounts can interfere with calcium absorption; this mineral is necessary to form bone tissue (with calcium) and is involved in many regulatory functions
Iodine	Many varieties of seafood, iodized salt, vegetables grown in iodine-rich soil	Iodine is a component of thyroid hormones, which control the body's energy metabolism
Magnesium	Legumes, milk, meat, seafood, nuts, eggs, whole grains, green leafy vegetables; hard water is an additional source of magnesium, although we rarely consume high amounts of hard water since the advent of filtered water	Magnesium is involved in muscle relaxation, protein synthesis, energy release, and calcium absorption

Continued overleaf

Table 9.1 Vitamins and Minerals, *continued*

Vitamin/Mineral	Source	Function
Zinc	Organ meats (e.g., liver), oysters, soybeans, spinach, whole grains	A component of several different enzymes that aid in the metabolism of foods; also a part of the hormone insulin
Copper	Seafood, eggs, legumes, meats, nuts, whole-grain cereals, raisins	Aids in iron absorption; also a component of enzymes that help form collagen and hemoglobin
Chromium	Whole grains, meats, cheese, eggs	While many supplement manufacturers claim chromium supplementation is generally beneficial in blood sugar control and/or fat burning, there is no good evidence for widespread chromium deficiency (there is only a marginal effect for those who may be deficient—primarily, some Type 2 diabetics); there is no set RDA for chromium as it is found in adequate amounts in whole grains, meats, cheese, and eggs; Chromium, which is part of glucose tolerance factor (GTF), regulates the metabolism of glucose in the body

Table 9.2 Recommended Daily Dietary Allowances (RDA) for for Protein and Fat-Soluble Vitamins

	Age (yr)	Weight (lb)	Height (in)	Energy (kcal)	Protein (g)	Vit. A (IU)	Fat-Soluble Vitamins Vit. D (IU)	Vit. E (IU)
Infants	Birth–6 mos.	14	24	117 per kg	2.2 per kg	1,400	400	4
	7 mos.–1 yr.	20	28	108	2.0	2,000	400	5
Children	1–3 yrs.	28	34	1,300	23	2,000	400	7
	4–6	44	44	1,800	30	2,500	400	9
	7–10	66	54	2,400	36	3,300	400	10
Males	11–14	97	63	2,800	44	5,000	400	12
	15–18	134	69	3,000	54	5,000	400	15
	19–22	147	69	3,000	54	5,000	400	15
	23–50	154	69	2,700	56	5,000		15
	over 50	154	69	2,400	56	5,000		15
Females	11–14	97	62	2,400	44	4,000	400	12
	15–18	119	65	2,100	48	4,000	400	12
	19–22	128	65	2,100	46	4,000	400	12
	23–50	128	65	2,000	46	4,000		12
	over 50	128	65	1,800	46	4,000		12
Pregnant				+300	+30	5,000	400	15
Lactating				+500	+20	6,000	400	15

Note: Vitamins mentioned in the text for which there is no RDA at this time include biotin and pantothenic acid. Minerals needed in only trace amounts include sodium, chlorine, potassium, sulfur, manganese, cobalt, and copper.

Source: Adapted from Food and Nutrition Board, National Academy of Sciences/National Research Council, in *The Type 2 Diabetes Diet Book* (Los Angeles: Lowell House, 1999).

Table 9.3 Recommended Daily Dietary Allowances (RDA) for Water-Soluble Vitamins

	Age (yr)	Ascorbic Acid (mg)	Folic Acid (mcg)	Niacin B_3 (mg)	Riboflavin B_2 (mg)	Thiamine B_1 (mg)	Pyridoxine B_6 (mg)	Cyanocobalamin B_{12} (mg)
Infants	Birth–6 mos.	35	50	5	0.4	0.3	0.3	0.3
	7 mos.–1 yr.	35	50	8	0.6	0.5	0.4	0.3
Children	1–3 yrs.	40	100	9	0.8	0.7	0.6	1.0
	4–6	40	200	12	1.1	0.9	0.9	1.5
	7–10	40	300	16	1.2	1.2	1.2	2.0
Males	11–14	45	400	18	1.5	1.4	1.6	3.0
	15–18	45	400	20	1.8	1.5	2.0	3.0
	19–22	45	400	20	1.8	1.5	2.0	3.0
	23–50	45	400	18	1.6	1.4	2.0	3.0
	over 50	45	400	16	1.5	1.2	2.0	3.0
Females	11–14	45	400	16	1.3	1.2	1.6	3.0
	15–18	45	400	14	1.4	1.1	2.0	3.0
	19–22	45	400	14	1.4	1.1	2.0	3.0
	23–50	45	400	13	1.2	1.0	2.0	3.0
	over 50	45	400	12	1.1	1.0	2.0	3.0
Pregnant		60	800	+2	+0.3	+0.3	2.5	4.0
Lactating		80	600	+4	+0.5	+0.3	2.5	4.0

Note: Vitamins mentioned in the text for which there is no RDA at this time include biotin and pantothenic acid. Minerals needed in only trace amounts include sodium, chlorine, potassium, sulfur, manganese, cobalt, and copper.

Source: Adapted from Food and Nutrition Board, National Academy of Sciences/National Research Council, in *The Type 2 Diabetes Diet Book* (Los Angeles: Lowell House, 1999).

Table 9.4 Recommended Daily Dietary Allowances (RDA) for Minerals

	Age (yr)	Calcium (mg)	Phosphorus (mg)	Iodine (mg)	Iron (mg)	Magnesium (mg)	Zinc (mg)
Infants	Birth–6 mos.	360	240	35	10	60	3
	7 mos.–1 yr.	540	400	45	15	70	5
Children	1–3 yrs.	800	800	60	15	150	10
	4–6	800	800	80	10	200	10
	7–10	800	800	110	10	250	10
Males	11–14	1,200	1,200	130	18	350	15
	15–18	1,200	1,200	150	18	400	15
	19–22	800	800	140	10	350	15
	23–50	800	800	130	10	350	15
	over 50	800	800	110	10	350	15
Females	11–14	1,200	1,200	115	18	300	15
	15–18	1,200	1,200	115	18	300	15
	19–22	800	800	115	18	300	15
	23–50	800	800	100	10	300	15
	over 50	800	800	80	10	300	15
Pregnant		1,200	1,200	125	18+	450	20
Lactating		1,200	1,200	150	18	450	25

Note: Vitamins mentioned in the text for which there is no RDA at this time include biotin and pantothenic acid. Minerals needed in only trace amounts include sodium, chlorine, potassium, sulfur, manganese, cobalt, and copper.

Source: Adapted from Food and Nutrition Board, National Academy of Sciences/ National Research Council, in The Type 2 Diabetes Diet Book (Los Angeles: Lowell House, 1999).

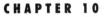
How To Succeed Immediately: The 1,000-Calorie, 35-Gram Carbohydrate Solution

By NOW, YOU KNOW THE BENEFITS of burning your fat stores. Ketosis, as explained earlier, is a very beneficial state in which insulin is effectively lowered and fat is released for energy. What follows are detailed descriptions of the 1,000-calorie and 35-gram carbohydrate diet, food lists, and sample menus for two weeks.

THE INSULIN CONTROL DIET

Daily Meal Plan

Breakfast

1 egg or 3 egg whites or egg substitutes *or* ½ cup cottage cheese *or* protein supplement drink

Sugar-free gelatin (optional)

Any sugar-free beverages, including coffee and tea

Midmorning snack (optional)

Vegetables from free food list, bouillon, dill pickles, sugar-free gelatin, any sugar-free beverages

Lunch

5 ounces protein (e.g., fish, chicken, *or* turkey)
Salad with free vegetables
Sugar-free beverages

Midafternoon snack (optional)

Vegetables from free food list, bouillon, dill pickles, sugar-free
gelatin, any sugar-free beverages
If needed (optional): 1 ounce cheese (e.g., string cheese stick) *or*
1 ounce other protein (e.g., turkey) *or* protein supplement drink

Dinner

5 ounces protein
Salad with free vegetables
½ cup cooked *or* raw vegetables
Any sugar-free beverages

Dessert

Sugar-free gelatin with whipped topping *or* sugar-free cocoa *or*
sugar-free ice pop

Additional optional foods

1 serving fruit *and/or* 1 serving starch
1 to 2 tablespoons whipped topping

Food List*

This menu provides for you a basic outline for your daily food
intake. The following food lists detail the amount of carbohydrate
per serving in each food group.

*Source: *The Type 2 Diabetes Diet Book,* 3d edition (Los Angeles: Lowell House, 1999).

Protein

(0–1 gram carbohydrate per serving) In general, serving sizes range from 3 to 5 ounces.

Fish: all varieties, fresh *or* frozen (e.g., salmon, halibut, orange
    roughy, etc.)
Shellfish: all varieties, fresh *or* frozen (e.g., shrimp, lobster, crab,
    scallops, etc.)
Poultry: chicken, turkey, Cornish hens (without skin)
Meat: beef (lean cuts, all visible fat removed)
    veal (leanest cut)
    pork tenderloin
    ham (labeled 95 percent fat free)
    Canadian bacon
Cheese: cottage cheese (nonfat *or* low fat)
    varieties of cheese (nonfat *or* low fat types)
    grated Parmesan
Eggs: whole eggs (omit yolk if cholesterol levels are high)
    egg whites
    egg substitutes
Other: tofu (soy)
    uncreamed herring

Vegetables

(5 grams carbohydrate per serving, ½ cup raw or cooked, unless otherwise noted) These vegetables are low in carbohydrates, are rich in fiber, and provide important vitamins and minerals.

artichoke, ½ medium	mushrooms, *cooked*
asparagus	okra
bean sprouts	onions
beans (wax, green, snap, Italian)	pea pods

broccoli
Brussels sprouts
cabbage (green, red), *cooked*
carrots, *raw*
cauliflower
eggplant
greens (collard, mustard, turnip)
kohlrabi
leeks

peppers (green, yellow, red)
rutabaga
sauerkraut
spinach, *cooked*
summer squash (crookneck *or* pattypan)
tomato: 1 large, *or* ½ cup juice
turnips
zucchini, *cooked*

Fruits

(15 grams carbohydrate per serving) Specific serving sizes are listed below.

apple, raw, 1 small
applesauce, unsweetened, ½ cup
apricot, raw, 4 medium
apricots, canned, ½ cup
   or 4 halves
banana, ½ medium *or* 1 junior
blackberries, raw, ¾ cup
cantaloupe, cubed, 1 cup
cherries, raw, 12 large
cherries, canned, ½ cup
figs, raw, 2
fruit cocktail, ½ cup
grapefruit, ½ medium
grapefruit segments, ¾ cup
grapes, 15
honeydew melon, cubed, 1 cup
kiwi, 1 large

mandarin oranges, ¾ cup
mango, ½ small
nectarine, 1 small
orange, 1 small
papaya, 1 cup
peach, 1 small *or* ¾ cup
peaches, canned, ½ cup
pear, ½ large *or* 1 small
persimmon, 2 medium
pineapple, raw, ¾ cup
plum, raw, 2 small
pomegranate, ½
raspberries, raw, 1 cup
strawberries, raw, 1¼ cups
tangerine, raw, 2 small
watermelon, raw, 1¼ cups

Starch

(15 grams carbohydrate per serving) Specific serving sizes are listed below.

Starchy vegetables

corn, ½ cup

corn on the cob, 6-inch ear

jicama, ½ cup

parsnips, ½ cup

peas, ½ cup

plantain, ½ cup

potatoes, ½ cup, 1 small

winter squash

  (acorn, butternut), ½ cup

water chestnuts, ½ cup

yams *or* sweet potatoes, ⅓ cup

Grains and pastas

bulgur, cooked, ½ cup

cornmeal, dry, 2½ tbsps

couscous, cooked, ⅓ cup

pasta, cooked, ½ cup

rice, cooked, ⅓ cup

wheat germ, 3 tbsps

millet, cooked, ⅓ cup

Cereals

bran flakes, ½ to ¾ cup

creamed wheat, cooked, ½ cup

oat flakes, ½ to ¾ cup

oatmeal, cooked, ½ cup

wheat flakes, ½ to ¾ cup

Bread and crackers

bagel, ½ small

bread, 1 slice

crackers, whole grain, 2 to 4

English muffin, ½

pita, 6-inch, ½

rolls, plain, 1 small

tortilla, corn, 6-inch, 1

Free Foods

If no serving size is specified, eat free foods in *moderation*.

Vegetables

cabbage, *raw*

celery

cucumber

dill pickles, 2–4

endive

green onion

hot peppers

lettuce (all varieties)

mushrooms, *raw*

radishes

spinach, *raw*

watercress

zucchini, *raw*

Sweets

extracts

sugar-free gelatin

whipped topping, 2 tbsps.

sugar substitutes (Equal,
Sweet 'N Low, stevia)

Hints

- stevia is a natural sweetener made from herbs
- sugar-free ice pops and cocoa provide 3–5 grams carbohydrate, check label

Drinks

club soda

cocoa powder (no sugar),
  1 teaspoon

coffee, decaf *or* regular

fat-free bouillon *or* broth

sugar-free drink mixes
  (e.g., Crystal Light)

sugar-free sodas

tea, decaf *or* regular

Miscellaneous

herbs

horseradish

soy sauce

spices

marinades (< 2 grams carbohydrate [CHO]/serv.)
nonstick cooking spray
butter substitutes, (e.g., "I Can't Believe It's Not Butter" spray)
salad dressings (< 2–4 grams CHO/serv.)
vinegar

Hints

- For more specific nutrient breakdowns for foods, see Appendix B. There are many books available that list all foods with respective carbohydrate grams. Some suggested authors are Barbara Kraus and Corinne T. Netzer.
- All carbohydrate amounts may vary according to serving size and/or specific products used. Always check labels.

Menus

The following section provides two weeks of menus that comply with the Insulin Control Diet. Each day provides roughly 35 to 40 grams of carbohydrate. Calories for each day are approximately 1,000 (800 to 1,200); however, these numbers may vary due to portion sizes and cooking methods. See Appendix A for complete recipes (given in italics) with respective calorie and carbohydrate breakdowns.

Week One
Day 1

Breakfast
1 egg, boiled
½ apple
sugar-free gelatin
coffee *or* other sugar-free beverage

Snack
bouillon

Lunch
tuna
large salad with free vegetables
1 slice whole-grain bread (low-carb variety)
sugar-free beverage

Snack
½ apple

Dinner
Skewered Sesame Chicken
½ cup steamed broccoli
small salad with free vegetables
sugar-free beverage

Dessert
sugar-free gelatin with 1 tablespoon whipped topping

Day 2

Breakfast
½ cup cottage cheese, nonfat *or* low fat
½ cup strawberries
beverage

Snack
sugar-free gelatin

Lunch
Turkey Roll-Ups

salad with free vegetables
sugar-free beverage

Snack
1 mozzarella string cheese stick
1 dill pickle

Dinner
Taco Chicken
large salad with free vegetables
¼ cup tomatoes, diced
¼ cup beans
sugar-free beverage

Dessert
½ cup strawberries
1 tablespoon whipped topping

Day 3

Breakfast
1 egg *or* 3 egg whites, scrambled
1 slice whole-grain toast (low-carb variety)
sugar-free beverage

Snack
1 small orange

Lunch
Scallop Ceviche
 served on endive
sugar-free beverage

Snack
2 dill pickles

Dinner
Tuna with Lemon and Sorrel
large salad
½ cup asparagus
sugar-free beverage

Dessert
sugar-free ice pop

Day 4

Breakfast
1 egg, poached
beverage

Snack
sugar-free gelatin

Lunch
Lean roast beef, sliced (from deli)
salad with free vegetables
1 small peach

Snack
bouillon

Dinner
Salmon Fillet with Dill and Leeks en Papillote
small dinner salad with free vegetables

½ cup steamed green beans
⅓ cup steamed rice

Dessert
sugar-free gelatin
1 tablespoon whipped topping

Day 5

Breakfast
½ cup cottage cheese
½ cup cantaloupe
beverage

Snack
sugar-free gelatin

Lunch
mesquite roasted turkey breast (from deli)
large salad with free vegetables
sugar-free beverage

Snack
1 *or* 2 dill pickles

Dinner
Grilled Swordfish with Red Pepper Salsa
small dinner salad with free vegetables
⅓ cup steamed rice
beverage

Dessert
sugar-free gelatin
¼ cup blueberries
1 tablespoon whipped topping

Day 6

Breakfast
chocolate protein supplement drink with less than 5 grams of
  carbohydrate per serving (e.g., Twinfast)
beverage

Snack
bouillon

Lunch
Pesto Chicken
salad with free vegetables
½ cup spinach

Snack
1 dill pickle

Dinner
Tofu and Portabella Stir-Fry
small salad with free vegetables
⅓ cup cooked couscous

Dessert
sugar-free gelatin
1 tablespoon whipped topping

Day 7

Breakfast
1 egg *or* 3 egg whites, scrambled
1 small nectarine
beverage

Snack
sugar-free gelatin

Lunch
Ranch Style Chicken
 diced
salad with free vegetables
¼ cup corn

Snack
bouillon
1 mozzarella string cheese stick (optional)

Dinner
Wine and Herb Beef
large dinner salad
½ artichoke

Dessert
sugar-free cocoa
1 tablespoon whipped topping

Week Two

Day 8

Breakfast
strawberry low-carbohydrate protein supplement drink
½ cup raspberries
beverage

Snack
sugar-free gelatin

Lunch
Halibut Brochettes
 served on endive, Boston, *or* Bibb lettuce
sugar-free beverage

Snack
bouillon

Dinner
Chicken with Sun-Dried Tomatoes
large dinner salad with free vegetables
Garlic Zucchini
beverage

Dessert
sugar-free ice pop

Day 9

Breakfast
½ cup cottage cheese
½ cup papaya, cubed
beverage

Snack
bouillon

Lunch
roasted turkey
free vegetables/salad
1 mozzarella string cheese stick

Snack
1 *or* 2 dill pickles

Dinner
Prosciutto Chicken
½ cup cooked pasta
¼ cup tomatoes
dinner salad with free vegetables
sugar-free beverage

Dessert
sugar-free gelatin
1 tablespoon whipped topping

Day 10

Breakfast
1 egg, boiled
beverage
sugar-free gelatin

Snack
½ small apple

Lunch
Grilled Scallops with Portabella Mushrooms and Feta Cheese
sugar-free beverage

Snack
bouillon *or* dill pickles

Dinner
Rosemary Pork Brochettes
small dinner salad with free vegetables
1 small potato

Dessert
sugar-free ice pop

Day 11

Breakfast
vanilla low-carbohydrate protein supplement drink (with
  flavored extract if desired)
beverage

Snack
½ small tangerine

Lunch
tuna
large salad with free vegetables
1 serving whole-grain crackers

Snack
dill pickle *or* bouillon
1 mozzarella string cheese stick

Dinner
Pignolas and Spinach Chicken
large salad with free vegetables
sugar-free beverage

Dessert
sugar-free cocoa
1 tablespoon whipped topping

Day 12

Breakfast
1 egg, boiled
sugar-free gelatin
beverage

Snack
bouillon

Lunch
Ginger Chicken Kebabs
   served with endive, Boston, *or* Bibb lettuce
sugar-free beverage

Snack
1 mozzarella string cheese stick (optional)

Dinner
Mahi-Mahi Stuffed with Veggies
⅓ cup steamed brown rice
small dinner salad
sugar-free beverage

Dessert
sugar-free gelatin
½ small orange, sliced
1 tablespoon whipped topping

Day 13

Breakfast
½ cup cottage cheese
½ small apple with dash of cinnamon
beverage

Snack
sugar-free gelatin

Lunch
Citrus Chicken
small salad with free vegetables
1 small roll

Snack
bouillon

Dinner
Poached Salmon with Vegetables
dinner salad with free vegetables
sugar-free beverage

Dessert
sugar-free ice pop

Day 14

Breakfast
chocolate low-carbohydrate protein supplement drink with iced
    brewed coffee
beverage

Snack
1 small plum

Lunch
Hot Shrimp
  served on endive, Boston, *or* Bibb lettuce
sugar-free beverage

Snack
1 *or* 2 dill pickles

Dinner
Almond Chicken
Herbed Mushrooms
⅓ cup cooked brown rice
small dinner salad with free vegetables

Dessert
sugar-free cocoa
1 tablespoon whipped topping

HINTS

- Any starches and fruits are optional. If you are not getting into ketosis, drop these options. You may be consuming too many carbohydrates.
- Why all the dill pickles and bouillon? You need salt! If you don't take snacks, add salt to your meals.
- By the way, snacks are optional.
- What's up with the gelatin? That, too, is optional. It is a nice filler and can help build strong nails and hair!
- Mayonnaise, butter, oils, and salad dressings should be used in limited amounts. While these foods have little or no carbohydrate, fat calories can add up.
- Remember: you can use salad dressings, herbs, and spices. Review your food lists.
- See Appendix A for recipes and suggested cooking methods.

CHAPTER 11

Support Strategies

A TYPICAL FIRST MEETING IN MY OFFICE goes something like this: Patients tell me that while they understand the principle of the diet, they fear they will struggle to lose the weight and will ultimately regain the pounds they have lost. They've tried every diet known to man with marginal success; yet, when all is said and done, the weight comes creeping back. Inevitably, they are left feeling like failures. Ketosis sounds like a safe and effective way to drop those unwanted pounds, but why should this time be any different? This is a valid concern; why should this program be any different? Simply put, it recognizes the need for support throughout the weight-loss phase and, ultimately, during stabilization and maintenance. While many of our readers do not have the benefit of working directly with a nutritionist, they can certainly utilize the many support strategies offered in this chapter.

The first question you need to ask yourself is why your previous attempts at weight loss were unsuccessful. Did boredom eventually lead to throwing in the towel? Maybe you felt deprived and found yourself bingeing on foods loaded with sugar and fat. Perhaps the weight loss was a breeze, but once the diet was over, all of those crazy cravings came creeping back . . . and the weight did, too. It is very important that you understand why losing weight and keeping it off may be difficult—and how to overcome that difficulty. Then, and only then, can you make the changes that allow you to successfully shed unwanted pounds and keep them off.

JOURNALING

I cannot overstress the importance of keeping a food journal during the course of weight loss. It invariably proves beneficial for a myriad of reasons. First, it holds you accountable to the diet. If you had four cookies, who is to say you actually did? Write it down! This in turn will provide a guide to your habits, difficulties with the program, areas of strengths, and areas of concern (e.g., difficulty eating out at lunch). Second, it is an account of how your body is responding to the program. Many times, patients have asked me why they are not achieving ketosis. There isn't a slice of bread to be found in their houses, yet their bodies just aren't budging. Writing down everything helps you to detect the hidden sources of carbohydrate/sugars in your diet that may be preventing ketosis. For example, you may be using a marinade, unaware that it contains sugar. Third, and perhaps most useful, you should record in your journal thoughts and feelings about the program and about certain foods in particular. How many times have you wandered to the refrigerator, opened the door, and taken something out to eat for no reason? You weren't hungry. What was going on?

I bet there *was* a reason. Journaling may help you see why you eat at certain times when you aren't really physiologically hungry. Maybe you were just bored. Perhaps you had a very stressful day at work or with the kids and felt you just "deserved a treat." Clearly, there is a physiological pull toward certain types of foods when you are feeling overwhelmed, upset, bored, and even happy; but, undeniably, there is another component. Many people are spurred to eat by emotions . . . not hunger. Write down these episodes, and what you were feeling. It will help you to pinpoint your most vulnerable moments and provide a guide to your eating habits so that changes can be made over time. For example, if you are aware that you are eating out of boredom, you can choose to participate in something else, such as exercise or other enjoyable activities. Figure 11.1 illustrates the use of a dietary journal.

Do you see any patterns in your own eating? Are there certain times of day when you feel the urge to munch? What foods do you tend to crave? If you are indeed snacking, what foods do you choose?

A WORD ABOUT TRIGGER AND BINGE FOODS

There are some things we just "can't get enough of." For many on this program, it is sugar: chocolate or death! For others, it is starchy foods; letting go of pasta seems unthinkable. Or perhaps it's fat—fried foods are like heaven. There is a physical reason you crave these foods; your body lets you know when it needs more serotonin. By eating certain foods, namely carbohydrate/sugar foods, you get a burst of serotonin. And you may feel great, but not for long. Your body soon demands more; thus you are trapped in a carbohydrate-craving cycle.

Why else do you crave certain foods for comfort? Perhaps when you were young, you were rewarded with a cookie when you were good. Over the course of years, you have associated good deeds with good foods. Whatever the scenario, the important point is that you do have a habit of eating certain types of foods when you are in certain moods. Once you start, it is hard to stop.

Claudette is a patient who loves chocolate. She has tried repeatedly to keep chocolate in the house because "her family enjoys it."

Figure 11.1 Dietary Journal

	Monday	Tuesday	Wednesday	Thursday	Friday	Saturday	Sunday
Breakfast	1 egg coffee sugar-free gelatin	½ cup cottage cheese coffee sugar-free gelatin					
Snack	Nothing	1 small apple					
Lunch	5 oz. turkey w/free veggies soda 1 bread	5 oz. shrimp, large salad ½ cup chilled asparagus tea					
Snack	1 string cheese	dill pickle (2)					
Dinner	5 oz. halibut ½ cup asparagus salad water, tea	5 oz. steak large salad, artichoke 1 tsp. mayo					
Snack	sugar-free gelatin ½ cup berries	whipped topping sugar-free cocoa					
carbs total grams	Approx. 35 g	Approx. 35 g					

Figure 11.1 Dietary Journal, *continued*

	Monday	Tuesday	Wednesday	Thursday	Friday	Saturday	Sunday	Notes
	Ketosis +/−	Ketosis +/−	Ketosis +/−	Ketosis +/−	Ketosis +/−	Ketosis +/−	Ketosis +/−	
	A.M.	A.M.	A.M.	A.M.	A.M.	A.M.	A.M.	
	P.M.	P.M.	P.M.	P.M.	P.M.	P.M.	P.M.	
	Exercise (yes/no)	Exercise (yes/no)	Exercise (yes/no)	Exercise (yes/no)	Exercise (yes/no)	Exercise (yes/no)	Exercise (yes/no)	
	Other: Good energy, not hungry, need more water (had about 50 oz.)	Other: water, great energy	Other: Increased	Other:	Other:	Other:	Other:	

Unfortunately, once Claudette allows herself one piece, she literally cannot stop. One piece of chocolate is never enough. Over time, Claudette has determined that she really can't have chocolate in the house; it is too difficult to abstain from eating it. By keeping this food out of the house, Claudette has controlled her sweet tooth, and has improved her weight loss along the way. Is there a trigger food for you? Can you eat just one cookie? Maybe the answer is no. Rather than taunting yourself on a daily basis, why not just eliminate these foods from your environment. Know your limits. Make a list. Be honest with yourself: What foods send you into a tailspin?

I can hear you already: "That's a great idea. I'd love to get rid of the pretzels and cookies, but I have a spouse who can eat anything she wants. My kids take this stuff to school. Why should I deprive them of these foods because I can't control my intake?" Fair enough. It might not be completely realistic for you to empty out the cupboards, but think about what you *can* do. If you are more aware of eating when you are not hungry, you can make an effort to substitute a different activity for the behavior. Rather than eating out of boredom, try to pick up a hobby or task that is meaningful to you. Another solution is to negotiate with your family. Perhaps you can all agree on snacks that are acceptable for your loved ones, but are not so appealing to you. Let your family members know how important their support is to you. Speaking of family and friends . . .

SUPPORT FROM YOUR FAMILY AND FRIENDS

Losing weight and keeping it off can be tough work; it requires many changes that must remain permanent. You don't want to revert back to your unhealthy past eating habits, but sometimes it's hard not to. We are a nation that revolves around food; we meet with our colleagues for lunch, we socialize after work with our friends at a local restaurant. After hustling to pick up our kids from soccer practice, we run through the drive-through. And need I mention how many holiday dinners we all attend with friends and family? I will make some suggestions on handling these social situations later, but first, let's start with the basics. Above all, it is critical to ask your friends and family for support—I bet they are willing to help.

Speak to your immediate family. Let them know that losing weight is important to you; it may very well be a matter of your health. A word to the wise: Do *not* expect your family members to take responsibility for your eating habits—only you can do that. You can expect understanding from your loved ones, however. Again, maybe your household can compromise on the snack foods in the cupboards. Frequently, I hear the following: "My husband brought home my favorite pastry from the bakery. He knows that I can't have it, but it's too hard to resist." The dieter then feels upset with herself for not sticking to the diet, and angry with her partner for "sabotaging" her diet. Once more, it is your responsibility to choose your foods wisely. Usually, the partner is just trying to please his or her loved one with a favorite treat. Unfortunately, it is once again the old idea of food as a reward. Talk to your loved one and let him know that you recognize the kindness of the gesture; however, it would be more helpful if he showed thoughtfulness through other methods, such as helping out around the house or picking up the kids.

Talk to your friends as well, and let them know that you would appreciate their support while you embark on the journey to weight loss. Perhaps, instead of meeting a friend for lunch, you can rendezvous at the park and take a walk. Try to spend time together doing things that are not centered on food. Clearly, we don't always have the time for such activities; however, making an attempt to change old patterns will certainly aid your effort to lose weight.

Holidays are a mix of emotional experiences, ranging from joy to pure stress! They're also a difficult time of year to cope with dieting. Friends and family, many of whom are not on diets, surround you. There is usually an abundant supply of goodies. Not only are there dinners with the standard fare, but there are often many holiday events, such as parties. Where does it end?

This is a common statement: "But Christmas comes only once a year. It is the only time we have (you fill in the blank)." True, Christmas, Hanukkah, New Year's, Halloween, Thanksgiving, Easter, Passover, Mother's Day, and Father's Day all come just once a year, but they'll be back next year, and the year after that. You may balk at the feeling that you might not ever eat a Christmas cookie or a latke ever again, but you can and will (on occasion, of course)! Be kind to yourself and remember that you have a goal. If you allow yourself to eat that cookie, will you stop at one—or will you set yourself up for uncontrollable cravings?

On the other hand, we recognize that sometimes it is just too difficult to avoid our favorite holiday foods. My suggestion is this: Allow yourself a small amount. You don't have to have large helpings. Yes, you will probably get thrown out of ketosis. You might even crave foods you haven't thought of in a while. Reconcile yourself to the fact that you chose to go off the diet for the day, accept it, and start fresh the next day. You can have a day off here and there, but proceed with caution! Thanksgiving is one day a year; it does not last Thursday through Sunday. Have small amounts of your favorite foods during the meal, and leave it at that. Don't eat leftovers all weekend!

Also, be realistic with yourself. Can you really allow yourself to go off the diet for one day and not feel guilty? Guilt is often the result of going off your diet, followed by more harmful eating and the "I'll start again on Monday" syndrome. Guilt is an unnecessary and counterproductive feeling! It will not help you stay in compliance with the program. Acceptance of your choices *is* important; understand that from time to time, we all slip back. This doesn't mean we can't continue to move forward and be successful in our attempts to shed unwanted pounds.

PRACTICAL TIPS FOR EATING OUT, HOLIDAYS, AND MORE

Dining Out

- Recognize portion sizes. Most restaurants serve large portions of protein (steak, chicken, fish). Ask for a take-out box and reserve half the meal. Of course, this is easier in certain situations.
- Split the meal with your companion. For example, order a main entrée such as fish or chicken with vegetables. Split this dish and supplement each portion with a dinner salad. This is a safe way to ensure smaller portions.
- Immediately ask your server to substitute additional vegetables for any starch. Don't tempt yourself unnecessarily.
- Ask how your meal is prepared. Ask that sauces be placed on the side. Remember: Grilling doesn't mean it is low-cal; it may have been grilled in butter.
- If possible, decline the bread basket at the beginning of the meal. Yes, this is difficult, but remember that one serving of bread is 15 grams of carbohydrate, on average. Most restaurant servings of bread are larger.
- At buffets, fill your plate first with protein and vegetables. If you absolutely must try something else, reserve only one-

quarter of your plate for extras. Don't go back for seconds. Make sure you get all the protein and veggies you need on the first go-around.

Holidays

Halloween

- Choose treats that are not food items. Pass out decorated pencils, special erasers, gift certificates, handy bottles of water, or other types of drinks.
- If candy is a must, choose one that isn't so tempting to *you*. Don't buy Snickers minis if they are absolutely your favorite.
- Give extra candy away. Neighbors, teachers, colleagues, and the like will appreciate the gesture.
- If you choose to take leftover candy to the office, be aware of temptation. Can you resist walking past the candy bowl? If not, ask a colleague to take the candy home.
- Thinking about sticking candy in the refrigerator? This, too, is a situation that leads to temptation.

Thanksgiving

- Attempt to eat only protein and vegetables. Stick to the obvious: turkey and veggies. Use the buffet rule. If you must experiment, reserve only one-quarter of your plate.
- Offer to bring hors d'oeuvres that are low-carb if you are attending someone else's dinner. For example, bring a platter of deviled eggs or a nice crudité with dip.
- Eat something early in the day. Starving yourself before dinner will only set you up to overeat out of hunger during the meal. Make a small dinner salad and have a hard-boiled egg or a piece of cheese before dinner.

- Drink plenty of fluids. Add a slice of orange or lime to seltzer water.
- If you choose to drink alcohol, recognize that alcohol contains empty calories and is not carbohydrate-free. Did you know that 4 ounces of wine provides roughly 4 grams of carbohydrate? Above all else, drink responsibly.
- One slice of pumpkin pie is approximately 35 grams of carbohydrate—that's an entire day's worth of carbohydrate grams. Opt for a low-carbohydrate dessert, instead.

Hanukkah

- One 3-ounce latke is 20 grams of carbohydrate and 190 calories. Traditional foods eaten during Hanukkah are laden with fat. Calories do make a difference.
- Again, stick to proteins and veggies only.

Christmas

- Many of the former rules still apply. Avoid any starchy foods and focus on filling up on dishes rich in protein.
- Drink sugar-free cider and cocoa for a festive treat.
- One slice of pecan pie is approximately 70 grams of carbohydrate and roughly 575 calories. I bet you'll think twice before taking that bite!

New Year's Eve

- Celebrations abound . . . and so does the endless supply of food. Try having a snack before any meal or party; this should help control appetite.
- If you choose to drink, drink responsibly. Champagne boasts approximately 5 grams of carbohydrate per 3 ounces.
- Rather than consuming alcohol, try drinking club soda with

a twist of lime, orange, or lemon. It's virtually calorie-free, definitely carbohydrate-free—and just plain safer.

Passover

- For ceremonial purposes, eat small amounts of carbohydrates (matzo). One piece of regular matzo is approximately 25 grams of carbohydrate.
- Don't be confused: just because a dessert is unleavened does not mean it is carbohydrate-free. While Passover foods are not made with wheat flour, many are made with potato flour. Potato starch is a big offender during the weight-loss phase.

Valentine's Day and Easter

- Chocolate! One piece of dark chocolate candy can have 9 grams of carbohydrate and 70 calories. Do you think it's worth it?

STAYING MOTIVATED

Now that you have an idea how to battle restaurants, parties, and holidays, it's time to address another very important issue. You have the strategies to stay on track, but what can you do to continue on your path to permanent weight loss? Staying motivated can be difficult, especially if you've been on the diet for extended periods of time. Clearly, weight loss in and of itself is a great motivator. Beyond this, it's important to find methods of encouragement and support that will allow continued progress.

ENLIST A BUDDY

If you have a friend, colleague, or spouse who needs to shed a few pounds, forge an alliance. Together, you can create new and lasting healthy habits. For example, make a date with your spouse or friend to go grocery shopping. You can compare shopping lists, help each other choose wisely, point out your favorite foods, and keep each other from making poor choices. Make exercising dates; there is no greater motivator for physical exercise than a companion. Compliment one another on your success, no matter how big or small. Every pound lost is an enormous achievement.

REWARD YOURSELF

Choose a specific amount of weight in pounds to be lost. For example, if you choose 5 pounds, reward yourself with something small each time an additional 5 pounds is lost. Give yourself a facial, go to a movie, buy a blouse, and so on. You don't have to spend money to reward yourself. Just doing something as simple as sitting in a hot bath without interruption or catching a sports game (or joining in one) can be very rewarding. Make a list of things that would be meaningful rewards specifically for you.

Rediscover an old love. Do you have an old hobby that you have long since abandoned? Why not rediscover the very things that bring you joy? Paint, read, build . . . play! Fill yourself up with activities that are enjoyable and—above all else—carbohydrate-free. Remember these gifts when you have the urge to eat unnecessarily. You will feel much better in the end because you chose to be kind to yourself and elected not to stuff your body with calories that would only make you feel worse.

One more pearl of wisdom: It is wise to be aware of your level of motivation. Simply put, sometimes we fall off track and have a hard time getting back on. By understanding your level of readiness to change, you can approach this program with more conviction. For example, if your spouse suggested that you begin this program, but you never really thought about losing weight, it might be difficult to follow the diet. On the other hand, if you have been thinking about shedding unwanted weight for some time, your level of commitment will be greater.

Dr. James Prochaska has created a very useful paradigm in which to discover one's readiness to change old habits. We progress through a series of stages commencing with precontemplation. In this case, precontemplation means that you haven't yet thought about going on a diet. If you've never thought about it or even recognized you have a weight problem, it will be quite difficult to stay on the program. The next stages are contemplation and preparation, during which you *think* about changing and you *prepare* to take action. Most of you are in the latter stage. You've picked up this book and are getting ready to start your journey. Beyond these stages, there are action, maintenance, and termination. In a nutshell, these stages entail making changes (big or small), working to maintain these changes, and—ultimately— achieving permanent behavioral change.

Dr. Prochaska, along with coauthors Drs. John Norcross and Carlo DiClemente, has also designed a very useful tool for creating lasting change. I recommend that you read more on this subject in *Changing for Good: A Revolutionary Six-Stage Program for Overcoming Bad Habits and Moving Your Life Positively Forward.*

This particular paradigm is only one way of approaching weight loss. I have found it useful when working with patients who have become "stuck" or have slipped back. These things happen, of course, to nearly everyone. It is helpful to get a sense of *why* they happen so that you can find appropriate solutions and move forward with success.

Above all else, remember that you had the good sense to pick up this book. By doing so, you have taken a major step toward better health. This makes you successful. Always remember that you are human and from time to time you might slip up; that's OK. Just do your best to get back on track. Ask for support; you deserve it. Always remember that the greatest gift you can give yourself is kindness. Don't beat yourself up if you aren't 100 percent perfect. *Everything* you do is a positive step toward success.

CHAPTER 12

Exercise: The Benefits of Aerobic and Resistance Activity

FOR MANY OF YOU, EXERCISE MAY BE an unknown. Your treadmill has conveniently become a clothes rack. The thought of lifting a weight is foreign. Maybe you once were active, but have become sedentary over time due to injury or illness. Perhaps you just don't think of the benefits of regular exercise and choose to involve yourself in different activities, like watching TV (sound familiar?).

Conversely, many of you might be regular exercisers. Perhaps you are looking for ways to improve on your current routine. Regardless of your level of fitness, exercise is indisputably an important component of permanent weight loss. Dieting by itself does *not* make for good health; it is only part of maintaining a healthy lifestyle. Exercise is essential, and the most expedient way to ensure that you keep off the weight you lose is to begin a regular fitness program. This chapter will discuss the benefits of cardiovascular exercise and address the value of weight training.

CARDIOVASCULAR EXERCISE

Cardiovascular, or cardiorespiratory, exercise involves using the large muscles of the body, during which time the lungs and heart work harder, resulting in improved aerobic fitness. There are many benefits from cardiovascular exercise. Regular exercise results in increased endurance, increased metabolism, lower blood pressure, improved cholesterol ratios, and improved glucose tolerance. Through regular activity, you can develop an increased ability to perform daily tasks with less fatigue, have more energy, and enjoy more restful sleep. This is only a small list of the many benefits of regular cardiovascular exercise.

While all these benefits sound appealing, the reality is that we often find it difficult to make time for exercise. Perhaps you are active now, but aren't sure how much consistent activity is necessary. There are many ways you can increase aerobic activity in your daily life without much effort. Before we explore this further, examine the following recommendations for cardiovascular exercise.

• RECOMMENDATIONS FOR •
CARDIOVASCULAR EXERCISE

- Exercise for a minimum of three days per week, building up to five days per week. If new to exercise, begin with a minimum of two days per week.
- Warm up for five to ten minutes before aerobic activity, including stretching.
- Exercise for a minimum of thirty minutes daily. This can be achieved by exercising for two fifteen-minute sessions or one thirty-minute session. Gradually increase duration of exercise to sixty minutes per session.
- Cool down for five to ten minutes, including stretching.

Source: Adapted from ACSM *Fitness Book*, 2d ed., Human Kinetics Publishers, 1992.

Don't be alarmed if your present activity doesn't fall within the guidelines. This is where you can begin to improve on your current regimen or get started. First, make a list of the activities you enjoy. It is always easier to stay fit if you are engaged in activities that are interesting to you. Here are some suggestions:

- walking
- treadmill
- jogging
- running
- biking
  (outdoors/stationary)
- hiking
- skating
- rollerblading
- swimming
- stair climbing (indoors/outdoors)
- rowing
- skiing
- sports (soccer, basketball,
  baseball, football)
- dancing
- kickboxing

Do any of these activities sound like fun? Some of these exercises may require a gym membership or home equipment. Walking, on the other hand, requires only you. This is perhaps the best activity for beginners (or anyone, for that matter). Walking has a blood sugar–lowering effect that is extremely beneficial. It is easy on the joints, yet it is extremely effective for building cardiovascular strength. For the purpose of this section, we will use walking as our exercise of choice.

GETTING STARTED

Let's suppose you are currently not active. It may be unrealistic to walk five days a week for thirty to forty-five minutes. Ask yourself how often you can walk at this time. Be realistic: Can you walk three days a week? Can you walk for thirty minutes? Maybe you can only walk for twenty minutes without stopping—that's OK. Let's start here, as an example. The objective, of course, is to reach a level of activity in your exercise program that is consistent with the listed recommendations.

There are four ways in which this can be accomplished. You can increase the *frequency* of your walks. If you are currently walking two days a week, add a third day. Try walking consistently three times a week for two to three weeks. Once this is part of your routine, try adding a fourth day, and so on. Another way in which you can modify your exercise program is to increase *duration*. If you are currently walking for twenty minutes at a time, after two to three weeks try adding an extra five minutes. Then, after walking for this length of time for a couple of weeks, add another five minutes, and so on.

If you feel you have reached your limit in terms of frequency and duration, you can choose to increase *intensity*. This might take extra effort on your part. If you have been walking at a slow to moderate pace, you might try increasing your pace for a portion of your walk. For example, walk slowly for the first ten minutes. Then, walk at a moderate pace for the following ten minutes, followed by an intense burst of energy for the third ten minutes. After slowly increasing your energy output over the course of weeks, you will be walking briskly for the duration of your walk. If you feel like you have reached the highest level of intensity, you might try adding ankle or handheld weights.

Beyond this, you might evaluate your exercise program and opt to add a different type of activity; you can change the *mode* of exercise. For example, if you have been walking five days a week for forty-five minutes at a moderate to high intensity, you might choose to add a different type of exercise to your routine. Ride a bike instead of walking, one day a week. Grab a group of friends and go for a hike instead of walking your usual route. By alternating your routine, you will remain interested in and excited about getting fit. Continue to build on your current routine; in a short time, you will be working out within the recommended guidelines.

TARGET HEART RATE

You can benefit from short bursts of physical activity as well as sustained cardiorespiratory activity. Generally, we can sense when our

---

• TARGET HEART RATE •

- 220 − age = estimated Heart Rate (HR)
- estimated HR × 60 percent = low end of HR
- estimated HR × 80 percent = high end of HR

Measure pulse at carotid artery (throat) by placing two fingers gently at pulse point. Count for ten seconds. Multiply number by 6. This number is your BPM (beats per minute).

Example: thirty-five-year-old, working at 80 percent

- 220 − 35 = 185 × 0.8 = 148 BPM (beats per minute)

---

bodies are working aerobically. Our heart rate increases and our breathing becomes heavier. As long as you can still talk to the person next to you, you are exercising at an appropriate intensity. If you are uncertain whether you are working within your target heart range, the following guideline will help you to determine your goal.

STAYING MOTIVATED

Just as teaming with a friend is helpful with the diet, so too is finding an exercise partner. If you are only accountable to yourself, you might make excuses to skip your workouts. If you have a friend with whom you exercise, you are more likely to stick to your routine. Make a date to go walking at the park or plan a hike together. Schedule appointments at the gym.

Speaking of scheduling appointments, many people are faced with working around busy schedules. How many of you use your work schedule as an excuse not to exercise? Too tired in the morning before you head off to work? Maybe by the time you leave the office, it's too late to go for a walk. Why not try scheduling activities into your day? Maybe walking at lunch isn't always feasible, but perhaps you can commit to two days a week. Schedule your exercise in your appointment book like any other important meeting. If the time is allotted for exercise activity, there are few excuses you can make. Consider it a commitment to your health.

Perhaps you can't imagine making time for even one workout—fair enough. Why not try to get in any amount of activity that you can? Did you know you can still benefit cardiovascularly from intermittent bouts of exercise? You can walk at a moderate intensity for ten minutes, three times a day, and still enjoy benefits. Almost everyone can afford to take a break sometime during the day. Take ten minutes to get some fresh air, or park farther from the office and walk the extra distance. Try using the stairs instead of the elevator. Park at the far end of the parking lot at the grocery store or mall and get moving! There are many ways in which you can fit in a few minutes of physical activity; it's up to you to make the choice. Remember that it is critical for weight-loss success.

WEIGHT TRAINING

Weight training, or resistance exercise, is an often-overlooked aspect of physical fitness; however, it is extremely beneficial for your overall physical health. Weight training results in increased capacity to perform work, bone mass, and fat-free mass (muscle)—which raises metabolism and motor performance. Risk of injury is reduced (it's easier to lift those heavy objects) and muscle strength becomes greater. Weight training can also result in small improvements in cardiorespiratory fitness, modest reductions in blood pressure, and improved glucose tolerance and blood lipid profiles.

Undeniably, one of its greatest benefits is the noticeable change in your physique. No, ladies, you will not develop bulging muscles like the bodybuilders you see on TV; hormonally, most women cannot support that type of tissue growth because they don't have enough testosterone. What you can expect is a small initial weight gain of approximately 2 to 4 pounds over a two-month period (men can expect the same, perhaps more). Don't fear this gain. Muscle is more compact than fat, pound for pound, so you should actually feel tighter and leaner. Weight training, or resistance exercise, is the best way to change the shape of your body.

Naturally, these changes cannot be achieved overnight. Just like cardiovascular exercise, muscle strength training is a gradual process that, over the long term, leads to major benefits both

---

**• RECOMMENDATIONS FOR MUSCULAR •
STRENGTH AND RESISTANCE TRAINING**

- Perform a minimum of one set per exercise. Multiple-set routines provide greater benefits.
- Complete ten to fifteen repetitions for each exercise. If new to exercise, or if you are an older individual, eight to ten repetitions are recommended.
- Perform at least three to four exercises for all major muscle groups.
- Perform these exercises a minimum of two to three days a week.

Source: Adapted from *ACSM Fitness Book*, 2d ed., Human Kinetics Publishers, 1992.

---

physically and psychologically. The above are the objectives of any weight-training program.

As with any exercise program, it is highly advisable that you consult your physician before you start. It is also recommended that you educate yourself on proper movement. Don't pick up a set of weights without learning how to execute each movement in a safe and effective manner. This might require you to enlist a trainer for a session or two. If this is not possible, you might refer to the *ACSM Fitness Book* for simple instructions.

FLEXIBILITY

In addition to achieving cardiovascular fitness and muscular strength, flexibility should be considered a fitness goal. Flexibility is defined as the range of motion possible around a joint or the ability of the tissues surrounding a joint to stretch and relax. The benefits of flexibility include decreased risk of injury, reduced stress, improved posture, relief of muscle soreness, and decreased lower back pain. It is advisable to stretch only after warming the muscles. Stretching is an excellent way to wind down your workout. Three to five stretching sessions per week are adequate for most individuals to maintain flexibility. For those attempting to gain flexibility, daily stretching is recommended.

PRACTICAL EXERCISE TIPS

Once you've started your exercise program, here are a few things to keep in mind as you continue working toward your fitness goals.

- Wear appropriate clothing. In warm weather, wear lighter clothes that allow your skin to breathe.
- Always wear comfortable shoes. Don't skimp on these; you don't want blisters slowing you down.
- Modify your pace (energy output) in warmer weather. Try exercising indoors. If you are outdoors, try to exercise in the morning or in the evening.
- Drink plenty of water. It is best to sip water throughout your workout, every fifteen minutes or so.
- Pay attention to any discomfort or pain. You may experience some stiffness or discomfort a day or two after starting to work out; this is normal, but pain isn't. If you are sore beyond a couple of days, you've strained your muscles. Be aware of how you feel during exercise. Is anything uncomfortable? Again, a new exercise program will be a challenge to your muscles, but you should not hurt!

- Keep an exercise log. It is highly motivating to be able to see your progress.

Always consult your physician before embarking on any exercise program, as recommendations may vary due to any medical limitations.

CHAPTER 13

Beyond Ketosis: Stabilization and Maintenance

YOU MADE IT! YOU HAVE REACHED your goal weight and now it's time to stabilize and maintain your successful weight loss. Stabilization is a critical aspect of this program. During this phase, you will learn how to slowly integrate carbohydrates into your diet.

It is important to follow the stabilization plan closely so your body will adjust to additional calories. Ultimately, you will determine the appropriate amount of calories and carbohydrates to maintain your current weight. By now you have hopefully developed an exercise routine that is both enjoyable and fits into your lifestyle. This, coupled with the maintenance diet, will ensure your long-term success.

STABILIZATION

The weight-loss phase of this program has now come to an end. Before you begin stabilization, be sure you have truly reached your goal; it is often easy to give up with those last 5 pounds still hanging on. You say to yourself, "I'll take off the last 5 pounds later. I'm ready to start stabilizing now." If this is the case, I suggest you rethink this plan. Keeping on the last few pounds will only make it easier to allow some weight gain beyond stabilization. Yes, you can always take it off again, but why not finish now? You deserve to reach your goal; you have made many changes and should be rewarded for them. Do yourself a favor and don't give up when you are so close to the finish line.

Stabilization is a critical component of this program. For some time now, you have restricted carbohydrates in the diet. You might not even crave these types of foods anymore. For variety and for balance, though, it is time to add some to your meals. It must be done slowly! Why is this so important? Following ketosis, the body isn't used to carbohydrates. If you rapidly reintroduce carbohydrates, the body will respond by retaining fluid; there might also be changes in digestion. You should anticipate a small amount of fluid retention, but nothing extreme. It is not unusual to experience 1 or 2 pounds of water retention; however, this should in no way deter you from reintroducing carbohydrates to your diet. Carbohydrates will provide you with beneficial fiber and other nutrients and will allow for more flexibility in your food choices. An easy-to-use chart for stabilization is provided at the end of this chapter.

At this point, you are most likely still in ketosis. You might even be losing weight beyond your goal. By adding a small amount of carbohydrate, the body will stop producing ketones; you can see this by measuring ketones in your urine with Ketostix. During the first week, it is recommended that only one serving of vegetable carbohydrates be added to the current diet. One ounce of protein should also be added. You can eat these additional foods at any time during the day. Make sure your fluid intake is consistent; now is not the time to quit drinking water!

It's possible you will still remain in ketosis and consequently drop a couple of pounds during the first week. If this is the case, you may add one serving of fruit. If your weight has stayed the same, add one additional serving of vegetable carbohydrates.

Again, add 1 ounce of protein. By now, you have made it through two weeks of stabilization. It's not so bad, is it?

During the third week, if you are still losing weight, add two servings of carbohydrate. This can be anything you want from the fruit, starch, or vegetable category. You can also add another ounce of protein if you choose. Keep up with your journal. It's important to track your daily intake. During the fourth week, you might start to maintain your weight. If this is the case, add one serving of carbohydrate (your choice). *Do not eat simple sugars.* If you gain, remove the serving of carbohydrate; it's that simple. If you aren't gaining, you may also add one serving of oil. (Be sure to read the section on "good" fats later in this chapter.)

During the fifth and sixth weeks of stabilization, you should continue your current intake of protein and carbohydrates. You might even try adding one serving of dairy in place of a carbohydrate or protein serving. Week seven and beyond are equally important. Continue to keep track of your intake as well as your weight. If your weight is staying the same, you have reached your maintenance level of carbohydrates. Now that you have a sense of what your maintenance program looks like, let's discuss the importance of the last phase.

MAINTENANCE

Now you are eating a more balanced diet and maintaining your hard-earned weight loss. Throughout your journey, you have made many changes in both your dietary and exercise habits. This is certainly not the time to revert to your old, unhealthy ways. Undoubtedly, you have gained the strength to maintain your new healthy status, but there are still some unanswered questions. How many calories should I be eating daily? What about fats and alcohol? What if I gain a few pounds? Can I ever eat sugar again?

It's important to understand how your maintenance level of calories is determined. In order to sustain your weight, your body demands a certain intake of calories at a resting state. If you are active, the calorie demand is higher. A bodybuilder who weighs 230 pounds will certainly need many more calories than a sedentary individual who weighs 120 pounds. An easy method of determining your calorie needs follows.

A balanced diet will provide approximately 30 percent of calories from fat, 40 to 50 percent of calories from carbohydrate, and 20 to 30 percent of calories from protein. One gram of carbohydrate is 4 calories, 1 gram of protein is 4 calories, and 1 gram of fat is 9 calories. The following example illustrates a 2,000-calorie diet composed of 30 percent fat, 40 percent carbohydrate (CHO), and 30 percent protein.

• CALORIES AND GRAMS FOR • FAT, CARBOHYDRATE, AND PROTEIN

30 percent fat of 2,000 calories = 600 calories @
9 calories per gram fat = 67 grams fat
40 percent carbohydrate of 2,000 calories = 800
calories @ 4 calories per gram CHO = 200 grams
carbohydrate
30 percent protein of 2,000 calories = 600 calories
@ 4 calories per gram protein = 150 grams protein

Examples

1 4-ounce piece of chicken (cooked) = 5 g fat, 0 g
carbohydrate, 30 g protein
1 cup milk (nonfat) = 1 g fat, 12 g carbohydrate, 8 g protein
1 slice whole-grain toast = 1 g fat, 13 g carbohydrate,
2 g protein
1 cup broccoli (steamed) = <1 g fat, 8 g carbohydrate,
5 g protein
1 tablespoon olive oil = 14 g fat, 0 g carbohydrate, 0 g protein

---

ALL FATS ARE NOT CREATED EQUAL

The amount of fat in your diet should be limited during the weight-loss phase; however, small amounts of dietary fat are permissible during stabilization and maintenance. One gram of fat equals 9 calories. It doesn't matter if it is butterfat or olive oil; per gram, it is the same. There is definitely a significant difference in the health benefits of certain fats, however. There is no evidence that certain fats that contain monounsaturated and polyunsaturated fatty acids can adversely affect cholesterol levels. Conversely, saturated fatty acids have a detrimental effect on your cholesterol levels and, ultimately, your cardiovascular health. Table 13.1 illustrates the differences among dietary fats. Choosing those high in monounsaturated fatty acids is your best bet.

A WORD ABOUT NUTS

Recently, there has been much publicity regarding the benefits of nuts in your diet. There are certainly some nuts that provide beneficial fats—but don't start snacking just yet. Although nuts can provide protein and minimal carbohydrate, they can contain approximately 14 grams of fat per ounce. This contributes to almost half the calories! Go ahead and enjoy your nuts, but be aware of the calorie content; it can add up quickly. Table 13.2 is a guide to the good and not-so-good nuts.

MISCELLANEOUS MUST-KNOWS

Without fail, patients ask about the use of alcohol during the weight-loss phase. There has been much news in the media about the potential cardiovascular benefits of small amounts of alcohol,

Table 13.1 Good Fats versus Bad Fats

Type	Calories	Fat (g)	Saturated (g)	Polyunsaturated (g)	Monounsaturated (g)
Oils* (per tbsp)					
Canola (rapeseed)	120	14	1	4	8
Olive	120	14	2	1.5	10
Safflower	120	14	1	11	2
Peanut	120	14	2	5	7
Sesame	120	14	2	6	6
Hazelnut	120	14	1	2	11
Almond	120	14	1	4	9
Vegetable	120	14	N/A	N/A	N/A
Solids (per tbsp)					
Butter†	100	11	7	N/A	N/A
Margarine‡	100	11	7	N/A	N/A
(Safflower)	100	12	2	4.5	2
(Soybean)	100	11	2	4	3
(Vegetable)	90	10	2	2	2.5

Note: Grams are rounded to nearest whole number.

*All oils are cholesterol-free.

†Butter contains 30 milligrams cholesterol per tablespoon.

‡Margarine is cholesterol-free.

Table 13.2 Nuts

Type	Calories*	Fat* (g)				Carbohydrate* (g)	Fiber* (g)
		Total	Saturated	Polyunsaturated	Monounsaturated		
Almond	170	15	1.5	3	10	6	3
Cashew	170	14	3	2.5	8	8	1
Filbert	180	18	1.5	1.5	14	4	2
Hazelnut	200	18	1	N/A	N/A	4	3
Macadamia	220	22	3	N/A	N/A	3	2
Peanut	170	14	2	4	7	6	2
Pecan	190	19	1.5	5	11	5	2
Pignola	150	14	2	6	5	4	1
Pistachio	160	14	2	4	8	5	3
Walnut	180	16	1.5	12	4	5	2

*Per ¼ cup

specifically wine. While this is true, the fact remains that alcohol provides 7 calories per gram—that is, more than a gram of carbohydrate and less than a gram of fat. Alcohol has no nutritive value, and it isn't carbohydrate-free. For example, a 4-ounce glass of wine has approximately 4 grams of carbohydrate. Beyond this, alcohol weakens one's resolve. Snacking on forbidden foods becomes easy after a drink or two. We advise that there be no alcohol consumption during the weight-loss phase. During maintenance, an occasional drink is fine. Until then, avoid drinking alcohol.

Another topic of interest is the use of sugar alcohol in food products. The packaging suggests that these food items are sugar-free, but don't be fooled. Once sugar alcohol (mannitol, sorbitol) is ingested, the body will break it down like sugar. Be savvy when it comes to shopping and always read the fine print. For more shopping ideas, see the shopping list in Appendix B.

STABILIZATION:
WEEKS ONE, TWO, THREE, AND BEYOND

Week One

- Add one vegetable carbohydrate serving to your current daily diet. This will add approximately 5 grams of carbohydrate to your meal plan.
- Add 1 ounce of protein to your current daily diet for a total of 9 ounces for women, 11 ounces for men.
- Consume eight to ten 8-ounce glasses of water daily.
- Keep your daily journal; include food intake and exercise.
- Weigh yourself periodically.

Week Two

- If you have not gained or lost weight during week one, add another vegetable carbohydrate (5 grams) to your current menu. If you have lost weight, add one fruit carbohydrate (15 grams).
- Add 1 ounce of protein for a total of 10 ounces for women, 12 ounces for men.
- Continue to exercise regularly. Is it time to increase either the duration or frequency of your workout?
- Keep your journal daily.
- Consume eight to ten 8-ounce glasses of fluid.
- Weigh yourself.

Week Three

- One more ounce of protein can be added to current intake for a total of 11 ounces for women and 13 ounces for men.
- If you are still dropping weight, add two servings of carbohydrate. You can add from any list including fruit (15 grams), starch (15 grams), or vegetable (5) grams.
- If you are maintaining your weight, add one carbohydrate serving of your choice.
- Are you keeping track of your total carbohydrate intake? Make a note in your journal.
- Keep drinking fluids. Stick to sugar-free beverages and, of course, water.
- Maintain physical activity.
- Weigh yourself to assess any loss or gain.

Week Four

- Add another ounce of protein if desired.
- Add an additional serving of carbohydrate (your choice). If you gain, eliminate your serving.
- Add 1 teaspoon of oil, such as canola (rapeseed) or olive, to your daily intake. Avoid this addition if you are gaining weight.
- Consume eight to ten 8-ounce glasses of fluids daily.
- Are you moving? Keep exercising.
- Journal your food intake and exercise routine.
- Reward yourself! You've done an amazing job so far.

Week Five

- If you are active and can afford the additional calories, add one more serving of carbohydrate. Watch your weight! You may be approaching your limit.
- You may have one serving of dairy in place of 1 ounce of protein. One serving is 1 cup of milk or nonfat yogurt.
- How many grams of carbohydrate are you consuming daily? Keep writing down your daily intake of foods.
- Continue drinking fluids.
- Avoid simple sugars. Remember: these types of carbohydrates are like poison. Will you crave more after your first bite?
- Weigh yourself periodically.

Week Six

- If your weight is fluctuating, refer to your journal. Are you consuming simple sugars? Are you exercising less? How many servings of fruit and starch are you currently eating? Adjust your dietary intake accordingly and be sure to keep up with your exercise program. Perhaps it is time to increase your physical activity.
- Continue to consume plenty of fluids.

Week Seven and Beyond

- Continue to watch your intake of carbohydrates. Add and subtract foods as needed to maintain weight.
- Continue to reward yourself frequently for your hard-earned success.
- Weigh yourself as needed. How do your clothes fit? Are they getting tighter? This, too, is a great gauge of your weight-loss maintenance.

CHAPTER 14

Doctor to Doctor: An Overview of Endocrinology

I AM FREQUENTLY ASKED, WHAT IS an endocrinologist? In practice, I deal with the diagnosis and treatment of a variety of disorders caused by an imbalance of hormones. These are chemicals produced by certain glands that deliver their products directly into the bloodstream, which distributes them to target tissues throughout the body. The endocrine glands are the pituitary, thyroid, parathyroid, adrenal, pancreas, and sex glands.

The pituitary, or master gland, regulates the function of three other glands; namely, the thyroid, adrenal, and sex glands. It also produces a growth-stimulating hormone and prolactin, a milk-producing agent. The pituitary is not independent, however. It is governed by the nervous system through complex controls that funnel through the hypothalamus, that portion of the brain that lies directly above the pituitary. Many years of research have shown that there is no relationship between ordinary obesity and pituitary disorders. In rare cases of hypothalamic disease, extreme overweight may occur because of uncontrollable appetite and decreased metabolism.

There is still the widely held mistaken belief that an underactive thyroid causes obesity. This is because thyroid hormones stimulate metabolism. Thyroid-deficient patients rarely gain much fat weight, though, even when the hormone lack is extreme. Most of their modest weight increase is from an accumulation of mucinous tissue that traps extra water. In these cases, thyroid hormone treatment brings a dramatic improvement in well-being as well as weight loss. Many patients, and some physicians, mistakenly blame overweight on insufficient thyroid hormone, even when the now-available sensitive and accurate thyroid tests are normal. Adding thyroid hormone in such cases risks accelerating osteoporosis, and it may also destabilize the electrical activity of the heart, producing dangerous arrhythmias.

The pituitary controls the adrenal cortex via adrenocorticotrophic hormone (ACTH), which stimulates the production of cortisol, a life-maintaining hormone. Cortisol is also involved in sugar metabism and, for this reason, has been termed a glucocorticoid to distinguish it from other adrenal steroids (e.g., sex steroids), some of which have major male hormone activity (androgens). These adrenal androgens are also stimulated by ACTH. Cortisol—but not the adrenal androgens—when increased, suppresses the secretion of ACTH. Conversely, if there is even a mild deficiency of cortisol, ACTH increases to restore cortisol to normal levels. If the production of cortisol is inefficient, sustained elevation of ACTH increases adrenal androgen production, leading, in women, to acne, increased facial hair, sometimes thinning of scalp hair, menstrual irregularities, and infertility. Such a disorder is known as virilizing adrenal hyperplasia. It is the result of a deficiency of certain critical chemicals (enzymes) that drive the production of cortisol to completion. In its rare, but most dramatic form, extra androgen in the female fetus produces pseudohermaphroditism. The newborn appears to be a male with underdeveloped external genital apparatus (undescended testes) and a penis that lacks its usually placed opening and is really an enlarged clitoris. A late-onset form of virilizing adrenal hyperplasia is relatively common, with adolescent acne and excessive facial hair being the most usual manifestations. Treatment of virilizing adrenal hyperplasia involves mild suppression of ACTH with a small dose of cortisol or its equivalent.

Thinking about the disturbed relationships in virilizing adrenal hyperplasia led me to understand the importance of insulin resistance in obesity. Insulin is the blood sugar–lowering hormone and is stimulated by a rising level of glucose (e.g., after a meal) so that excursions of blood sugar are confined to a limited normal range. Insulin exerts its major effects on muscle, the liver, and fat. Insulin is not only the blood sugar–lowering hormone of the body; it also is the major fat-building, fat-storing hormone. Also, the release of stored fat is inhibited by small amounts of insulin. Insulin is also a powerful salt- and water-retaining hormone secondary only in importance to the adrenal hormone, aldosterone. As we have seen, insulin resistance in obesity does not involve all of these actions equally.

My first experience with insulin resistance was in diabetic patients who developed an increasing need for insulin to control their blood sugars. This was in the era of animal insulins, when we used beef or pork insulin for routine treatment. Doses of insulin were usually 40 to 80 units daily, and some patients appeared to require over 200 units to bring their blood sugars to reasonable levels. Some developed hives from their injections, suggesting the possibility of allergy. With the considerable help of Dr. Peter Moloney, an immunologist at the Connaught Laboratories in Toronto, I learned that these patients had produced an insulin-binding and neutralizing antibody that blocked insulin's blood sugar–lowering effect. This was demonstrated by the ability of the patient's serum to protect fasting mice from convulsions ordinarily induced by an established dose of insulin. Repeated testing with increasing dilutions indicated how much antibody was present in the serum.

At that time, Drs. Solomon Berson and Rosalyn Yalow were developing the Nobel Prize–winning technique of radio immunoassay (RIA), using insulin as a model substance to measure very small circulating amounts. When they came to Toronto as guest lecturers I introduced them to Dr. Peter Moloney, who agreed to provide some human insulin prepared at Connaught Laboratories to allow them to complete their studies. With the aid of their powerful tool, measuring insulin levels in the blood of diabetics revealed two major types of the disorder. In the young, thin diabetics, designated Type 1, there was little or no insulin to be found when the diagnosis was made. The other, much more common type of diabetes, occurring mainly in the older age group, had normal or increased levels of insulin to which the body was not responding in a normal fashion. This Type 2 diabetes appears to involve an insulin-resistant state with a component of decreased insulin reserve, limiting the capacity of the pancreas to increase insulin production enough to compensate for the resistance. Because most Type 2 diabetics are overweight, a question arose as to whether excess weight itself could be responsible for insulin resistance.

Subsequent studies have shown that obesity is invariably associated with a type of insulin resistance that is different from the insensitivity present in Type 2 diabetics who are not overweight. Recent research has shown that small amounts of tumor necrosis factor alpha (TNF-alpha), made in fat tissue and released into the circulation, is likely responsible for the insulin resistance in obesity. With loss of weight, TNF-alpha levels in the blood are correspondingly reduced. It is now established that obesity is associated with insulin resistance resulting in excess insulin production (compensatory hyperinsulinemia) to maintain normal blood sugar levels.

But what if there are other actions of insulin that are not affected by the resistance to its blood sugar–lowering effect? Indeed, there are. Two of the most important are insulin's effects on fat and its salt- and water-retaining action on the kidneys. Insulin is the fat-building and fat-storing hormone. Under insulin's appetite-stimulating influence, increased intake of predominantly carbohydrate calories is transformed into triglycerides that transport the storage form of fat to fat cells. Fat breakdown, to release this stored energy, is inhibited by insulin. The compensatory hyperinsulinism present in obesity contributes to further weight gain, predominantly from fat, but also due to some fluid retention, particularly in women. With increased fat weight there is more insulin resistance from TNF-alpha.

In obesity, the most important side effect of insulin resistance is excessive buildup of further fat. There are also a number of other systems that are less dramatically targeted for excessive stimulation from compensatorily increased levels of insulin. There are other sites of resistance to insulin action that produce further adverse effects as well. A notable example is the aggravation of hypertension by insulin resistance, which appears to be largely, but not solely, due to interference with the normal relaxing effect of insulin on arterial smooth muscle. Thus, insulin resistance in obesity produces a complex mixture of too much and too little insulin influence. What matters most, however, is the beneficial effect of reduction of insulin from a low-carbohydrate diet and increased aerobic exercise. There are now growing numbers of medications available to physicians that decrease insulin resistance and act cooperatively with the nondrug approach that we have just described. The most conservative approach should be tried first and only then should medication be employed, if necessary, to produce a more satisfactory result.

THE TWO THREADS OF DIABETES AND ENDOCRINOLOGY: SHOULD THEY BE JOINED?

Traditionally, diabetes and endocrine disorders have been regarded as separate conditions requiring different specialties for their investigation and treatment. From this concept, two specialty organizations have developed in this country: the American Diabetes Association and the Endocrine Society. While there has been some overlap in membership and program content at their respective scientific meetings, there remains a considerable disconnection between their scientific and clinical practice activities. In my lifetime, I have been fortunate to work in both diabetes and endocrinology simultaneously. From this ongoing crossfertilization have come some of my best ideas. The selective insulin resistance concept so important in our treatment of obesity arose from a series of observations. These began with the recognition that the blood sugar–lowering effect of insulin could be blocked by circulating antibodies because the insulin was held in the circulation by these antibodies and prevented from getting to its place of action on the surface of the cell. Therefore, all of its effects are equally inhibited. When we learned from the Nobel Prize–winning work of Berson and Yallow on radio immunoassay of insulin that Type 2 diabetes and obesity were insulin-resistant states, I wondered if obesity might be the result of a differential resistance to the blood sugar–lowering effect and compensatory fat-building hyperinsulinemia. An example of increased adrenal androgen production in virilizing adrenal hyperplasia that was the consequence of decreased production of cortisol provided a credible and relevant model that could explain what was happening in obesity. The adrenal androgen excess was being driven by oversecretion of the pituitary hormone adrenocorticotropic hormone (ACTH). When this was reduced by a small amount of cortisol-like medication, the androgen excess was corrected. The buildup of fat in obesity was being largely driven by excess insulin. It seemed reasonable to reduce the fat-building insulin with a low-carbohydrate diet and aerobic exercise, which have remained the mainstays of our insulin control program to this day.

Although there remain considerable practical difficulties in fusing the two specialties of endocrinology and diabetes, there is a welcome trend in this direction, particularly on the part of endocrinologists who now feel that with the availability of an array of new medications to treat diabetes, it is time for them to get more involved in managing these patients.

SUMMARY

There are many different kinds of insulin resistance. Most of them are the result of unknown abnormalities that lie beyond the insulin receptor that is found at the cell surface. Insulin resistance is defined by the defect in its blood sugar–lowering ability. There is a wide network of other insulin-acting sites that may continue to function normally and therefore be exposed to excessive insulin action in the presence of compensatory hyperinsulinemia. In insulin-resistant states, a rising blood sugar is met by an increased secretion of insulin, which restores the blood sugar to normal; however, at the same time, it may exert powerful additional effects throughout the insulin-responsive network. This relationship is the key to understanding the many varied manifestations of hyperinsulinism.

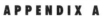

Recipes

DIETING DOESN'T NEED TO BE A DRAB, unexciting process. The following recipes all fall within the parameters of the Insulin Control Diet, without sacrificing taste. Although it may take extra time to prepare these meals, eating food that is enjoyable yet low in carbohydrate and sugar will help keep you motivated to follow the diet. You will probably enjoy some of these recipes so much that you'll make them permanent additions to your culinary repertoire!

RECIPE TIPS AND SUBSTITUTIONS

Miscellaneous Must-Knows

- Calories and carbohydrate grams may vary due to portion sizes and cooking methods.* Some recipes do not specify amounts for protein; calorie content may vary accordingly. Rule of thumb—3 ounces is roughly the size of a deck of cards.
- If oil is used in a marinade, you can reduce the amount. The marinade will appear thicker, but will contain less fat.

*Sources for calculation of carbohydrate and calories:
Calories and Carbohydrates, B. Kraus (New York: Penguin, 1997).
The Complete Book of Food Counts, C. Netzer (New York: Dell, 1991).

Remember—1 tablespoon of oil has 120 calories fat (14 grams).

- Cooking with oil is optional. You can use nonstick cooking sprays on grills and in skillets. This, too, will alter calorie content.
- Many of these recipes can be prepared using various cooking methods. Poultry, beef, and firm fish all cook nicely on the grill.
- Many of the marinades and/or seasonings are just as tasty with other types of protein. Experiment. Try some of the recipes with tofu. You'll be pleasantly surprised.
- Don't be afraid to try additional herbs and spices. You don't have to follow recipes exactly. If you like a little more spice, add some! For recipes with chili peppers, be aware that the seeds have the heat. If you like the "burn," keep the seeds.

Substitutions

- Instead of using butter, margarine, or oils, try using equal parts liquid in recipes (wine, stock, water, or other liquids).
- If marinades call for sugar, try using a substitute sweetener:

  1 packet of Equal = 2 teaspoons sugar
  ⅓ teaspoon Sweet 'N Low = 1 tablespoon sugar

VEGETABLES

Cauliflower, Mushroom, and Onion Bake

3   cups cauliflower

1¼ cup chopped mushrooms
½ cup chopped red onion
1   tablespoon olive oil
2   teaspoons lemon juice
2 to 3 teaspoons cider vinegar (depends on desired tartness)
½ teaspoon salt
⅓ teaspoon pepper
2   large cloves garlic, finely chopped
½ cup chopped green onions

Heat oven to 350 degrees. Spray baking dish with nonstick cooking spray. Mix all ingredients, reserving green onions. Spread evenly in dish. Bake uncovered 40 to 45 minutes. Sprinkle with onions.

Serves 6 • Calories 40 • Carbohydrate grams 5

Cucumber and Tomato Salad

2   medium tomatoes, cut into small wedges
2   cups sliced cucumber
¼ cup green onions
½ teaspoon dried dill
½ teaspoon regular powdered fruit pectin
¼ teaspoon garlic salt
dash coarsely ground pepper
1½ tablespoons white wine vinegar

In mixing bowl, mix vinegar, pectin, dill, salt, and pepper. Toss with tomatoes, cucumbers, and onions. Chill 4 hours.

Serves 4 • Calories 20 • Carbohydrate grams 5

Garlic Zucchini

    4 large zucchinis
    1 tablespoon garlic powder
    4 tablespoons Parmesan cheese

Cut each zucchini lengthwise into two pieces. Spray nonstick cooking spray on baking pan. Place zucchini skin-side down. Sprinkle with garlic powder and Parmesan cheese. Broil 6 to 7 inches from heat.

Serves 4 • Calories 40 • Carbohydrate grams 5

Gazpacho

    1 green bell pepper, diced
    1 red bell pepper, diced
    1 large cucumber, quartered lengthwise and chopped (peel if desired)
    1 large tomato
    6 radishes
    3 tablespoons chopped fresh dill
    ¾ to 1 cup crushed tomatoes
    2 tablespoons lemon juice
    1 teaspoon chili powder (more if desired)
    salt and pepper, to taste

Layer vegetables in large serving bowl. Do not mix. Mix remaining ingredients in small bowl. Drizzle over vegetables.

Serves 4 to 6 • Calories 35 • Carbohydrate grams 7

Green Beans with Pancetta Bacon

    1½ pounds green beans, trimmed
    5 ounces pancetta *or* lean bacon, diced

⅓ to ½ cup minced shallots
1½ tablespoons rosemary, dried
2 tablespoons olive oil
2 to 3 tablespoons lemon juice

Cook beans in large pot until crisp-tender. Rinse with cold water. Set aside. In heavy skillet, cook pancetta or bacon. Transfer to towels. Reserve 1½ tablespoons fat in skillet. Add shallots and rosemary. Cook over medium heat for about 2 minutes. Add beans and stir. Add oil and lemon juice. Cook until beans are heated through. Season with salt and pepper. Sprinkle with pancetta.

Serving size: ½ cup (about 6) • Calories 50 • Carbohydrate grams 5

Herbed Mushrooms

4 cups mushrooms, halved
⅓ cup sliced white onion
⅔ cup dry white wine
½ teaspoon basil, dried
salt and pepper to taste
1 tablespoon parsley

In large saucepan, add onions to small amount of boiling water. Cook for 1 minute. Add mushrooms and cook for 1 minute. Drain water. Set aside.

In saucepan, add remaining ingredients, reserving parsley. Bring to boil. Simmer, uncovered, for 5 minutes. Add mushroom and onion. Chill for 4 to 24 hours, covered. Serve with sprinkle of parsley.

Serves 6 • Calories 35 • Carbohydrate grams 3

Sesame Asparagus Salad

1 pound asparagus, cut into 2-inch pieces
3 tablespoons cider vinegar
3 tablespoons soy sauce
1½ tablespoons sugar
2 teaspoons sesame oil
pepper or hot sauce, to taste
1 tablespoon sesame seeds

Steam asparagus over boiling water for 3 to 4 minutes, or until tender. Remove asparagus and rinse with cool water. Set aside.

Combine remaining ingredients, reserving sesame seeds, in small bowl. Mix well. Pour over asparagus. Chill.

Serves 6 • Calories 40 • Carbohydrate grams 6

Spicy Eggplant, Pepper, and Tomato Salad

1 1-pound eggplant
2 tablespoons olive oil
1 red bell pepper, roasted and diced (use ½ cup store bought)
2 medium zucchini, sliced ½-inch thick
2 cloves garlic, crushed
2 large plum tomatoes, peeled and diced
½ teaspoon crushed red pepper
1 cup water
1 green bell pepper, cut into ½-inch pieces
12 Kalamata olives, diced

Salt eggplant. Drain for 30 minutes. Pat dry and cut into ½-inch pieces. Heat oil in large skillet. Combine eggplant, zucchini, garlic, tomatoes, and crushed red pepper flakes in skillet. Add water. Bring to boil. Reduce heat and simmer for 15 minutes. Add peppers and simmer for 30 minutes. Add olives.

Serves 6 • Calories 85 • Carbohydrate grams 6

POULTRY

Almond Chicken

4   boneless, skinless chicken breasts
salt and pepper to taste
2   tablespoons butter
½   cup slivered almonds
⅓   cup chopped shallots
⅛   teaspoon ground nutmeg
½   cup dry white wine
½   cup chicken broth

Season chicken with salt and pepper. Melt 1½ tablespoons butter in large skillet. Add chicken breasts. Cook for 6 minutes, turning 1 to 2 times. Remove chicken and set aside. Add remaining butter. Add almonds and shallots. Cook for 2 to 3 minutes. Place over chicken. Add remaining ingredients. Bring to boil for 2 to 3 minutes. Spoon over chicken.

Serves 4 • Calories 280 •
Carbohydrate grams 2 (nuts add 50 calories per serving)

Cajun Chicken

4 boneless, skinless chicken breasts
cajun spice to taste

Season chicken breasts. Place on hot grill. Cook for 12 to 15 minutes or until chicken is done. Serve on bed of greens.

Serves 4 • Calories 200 • Carbohydrate grams 1

Chicken with Sherry, Soy, and Ginger

4 boneless, skinless chicken breasts
1 teaspoon olive oil or nonstick cooking spray
2 to 3 tablespoons soy sauce
1½ tablespoons dry sherry
1 tablespoon canola oil (or sesame oil)
1 teaspoon garlic, minced
½ teaspoon gingerroot, minced (⅛ to ¼ teaspoon powdered)
pepper to taste

Mix all ingredients together except chicken. Marinate chicken breasts for 30 minutes. Add 1 teaspoon oil to large skillet. Add chicken breasts and sauté over medium heat for 4 to 5 minutes on each side. For grilling or broiling, cook 10 to 12 minutes turning once, or until chicken is done.

Serves 4 • Calories 180 • Carbohydrate grams 1

Chicken with Sun-Dried Tomatoes

4 boneless, skinless chicken breasts
1 teaspoon olive oil or nonstick cooking spray
¼ cup sun-dried tomatoes, diced
2 tablespoons olive oil

1 tablespoon lemon juice
2 teaspoons garlic, minced
½ teaspoon thyme
½ teaspoon basil, dried
pepper to taste

Mix all ingredients together except chicken. Add chicken and marinate for 30 minutes. Add 1 teaspoon oil to large skillet. Add chicken and sauté over medium heat for 4 to 5 minutes on each side. For grilling or broiling, cook 10 to 12 minutes, or until chicken is done, turning once.

Serves 4 • Calories 225 • Carbohydrate grams 5

Chinese Plum Chicken

4 boneless, skinless chicken breasts
1 teaspoon olive oil or nonstick cooking spray
¼ cup Chinese plum sauce (purchased)
3 tablespoons rice vinegar, unsweetened
½ teaspoon Dijon mustard
1 teaspoon garlic, crushed
red pepper flakes, to taste

Mix all ingredients together except chicken. Marinate chicken in plum sauce mixture for 20 minutes. Add 1 teaspoon oil or nonstick cooking spray to large skillet. Add chicken and sauté over medium heat for 4 to 5 minutes on each side. For grilling or broiling, cook 10 to 12 minutes, until chicken is done, turning once.

Serves 4 • Calories 175 • Carbohydrate grams 3

Citrus Chicken

4   boneless, skinless chicken breasts
2   tablespoons lime juice
2   tablespoons orange juice
1   tablespoon shallots, minced
¼   teaspoon dried basil
¼   teaspoon oregano
salt and pepper to taste
1   tablespoon olive oil

Mix lime and orange juices with olive oil. Place chicken breasts in glass pan. Cover chicken with marinade. Sprinkle shallots, basil, and oregano over chicken. Marinate for at least 20 minutes. Bake chicken at 375 degrees for 30 to 35 minutes, or until chicken is done. Chicken can also be grilled. Grill for 10 to 12 minutes, turning once. For thicker breasts, cooking time may be longer.

Serves 4 • Calories 220 • Carbohydrate grams 3

Ginger Chicken Kebabs

1   pound chicken, cubed
2   tablespoons gingerroot, grated
2   cloves garlic, minced
2   teaspoons sesame oil
juice of 1 lime
wooden skewers (soaked in water for 30 minutes)

Toss all ingredients except chicken. Thread chicken pieces onto skewers. Place on hot grill. Cook for 8 to 12 minutes, turning once or twice.

Serves 4 • Calories 200 • Carbohydrate grams 2

Grilled Chicken with Citrus and Ginger

4 boneless, skinless chicken breasts
1 teaspoon oil or nonstick cooking spray
¼ cup orange juice
1 tablespoon lemon juice
1 tablespoon soy sauce
1 tablespoon gingerroot, minced (½ to ¾ teaspoon powdered)
1 teaspoon garlic, crushed

Mix all ingredients except chicken. Marinate chicken breasts in orange-ginger sauce for 30 minutes. Add oil or nonstick cooking spray to large skillet. Add chicken breasts and sauté over medium heat for 4 to 5 minutes on each side. For grilling or broiling, cook for 10 to 12 minutes or until chicken is done, turning once.

Serves 4 • Calories 200 • Carbohydrate grams 4

Italian Chicken

4 boneless, skinless chicken breasts
½ cup Italian dressing

Coat chicken with dressing, covering both sides. Place on hot grill. Cook 12 to 15 minutes or until chicken is done. Serve on bed of greens.

Serves 4 • Calories 220 • Carbohydrate grams 2

Pesto Chicken

4   boneless, skinless chicken breasts
1   cup fresh basil
¼   cup pine nuts
1½ teaspoons minced garlic
⅛   teaspoon black pepper
2   tablespoons nonfat plain yogurt
2   tablespoons olive oil
2   tablespoons white wine vinegar
black pepper to taste

Blend basil, pine nuts, 1 tablespoon olive oil, garlic, and pepper in blender. Add yogurt, 1 tablespoon oil, and vinegar. Warm over low heat. To cook chicken, grill or broil for 10 minutes, turning once. If using thicker breasts, cooking time may be longer. Check for doneness. Serve chicken with pesto sauce.

Serves 4 • Calories 275 • Carbohydrate grams 3

Pignolas and Spinach Chicken

4   boneless, skinless chicken breasts
1   pound spinach
2   tablespoons olive oil
2   tablespoons pignolas (pine nuts)
½   cup roasted red peppers (store bought)
salt and pepper to taste
2   tablespoons Parmesan cheese (optional)

Wash spinach thoroughly. Chop into small pieces. Heat 1 teaspoon oil in large skillet. Add spinach and cook until wilted. Add pine nuts, salt, and pepper. Cook for 4 minutes. Remove from skillet. Heat remaining oil. Add chicken. Brown both sides for

5 to 7 minutes total. Add spinach and pignola mixture. Sprinkle diced red peppers on top. Sprinkle with Parmesan cheese if desired.

Serves 4 • Calories 190 • Carbohydrate grams 5

Prosciutto Chicken

    4   boneless, skinless chicken breasts
    ¾   teaspoon sage, dried
    salt and pepper to taste
    2   tablespoons oil
    2½ ounces prosciutto
    3   ounces Mozzarella cheese, thinly sliced
    ½   cup dry white wine

Season chicken with salt, pepper, and sage. Heat oil in pan. Add chicken and cook 3 minutes until brown on one side. Turn once. Layer with prosciutto and cheese. Add wine. Reduce heat to medium-low and cover. Cook until chicken is white throughout and cheese is melted, about 3 minutes.

Serves 4 • Calories 240 • Carbohydrate grams 1

Ranch-Style Chicken

    4   boneless, skinless chicken breasts
    ½   cup ranch dressing

Cover chicken breasts with ranch dressing, coating both sides. Place on hot grill. Cook for 12 to 15 minutes or until chicken is done. Serve on bed of greens.

Serves 4 • Calories 220 • Carbohydrate grams 2

Rosemary and Garlic Chicken

4   skinless, boneless chicken breasts
1   teaspoon olive oil or nonstick cooking spray
2   tablespoons lemon juice
½   teaspoon rosemary, crushed
½   teaspoon crushed red pepper (use more for more heat)
¾   teaspoon cracked black pepper
4   cloves garlic, crushed
2   teaspoons olive oil

Flatten chicken breasts with a rolling pin. Combine lemon juice, 1 teaspoon olive oil, rosemary, crushed red pepper, black pepper, and garlic. Marinate chicken breasts for at least 30 minutes. Add 1 teaspoon oil to large skillet. Add chicken breasts and sauté over medium heat for 4 to 5 minutes on each side. For grilling or broiling, cook 10 to 12 minutes or until chicken is done, turning once.

Serves 4 • Calories 210 • Carbohydrate grams 2

Spicy Steamed Chicken with Vegetables

4   boneless, skinless chicken breasts
½   teaspoon salt
1   clove garlic
1 to 2 teaspoons ground coriander
½   teaspoon cumin
½   teaspoon red pepper flakes
black pepper to taste
1   medium carrot
1   cup broccoli florets
1   cup bok choy

Add water to steamer pot to 1 inch. Place rack in pot for steaming. Cover and bring water to boil. Cut chicken into 1-inch strips. Place in heatproof dish. Add rest of ingredients except broccoli and bok choy. Cover and steam for 10 to 12 minutes or until chicken is barely pink. Add remaining vegetables and steam for additional 8 minutes or until vegetables are tender-crisp.

Serves 4 • Calories 180 • Carbohydrate grams 6

Taco Chicken

4   boneless, skinless chicken breasts
taco seasoning mix (store bought)

Season chicken with taco mix. Place on hot grill. Cook for 12 to 15 minutes or until chicken is done. Serve on bed of greens.

Serves 4 • Calories 200 • Carbohydrate grams 1

3-Pepper Chicken

4   boneless, skinless chicken breasts
1⅓ tablespoons olive oil
1   red pepper, cut into small strips
1   green pepper, cut into small strips
1   yellow pepper, cut into small strips
1   small red onion, cut into small strips
¼   cup lemon juice
2   teaspoons fresh rosemary, minced (½ teaspoon dried)
1   clove garlic, pressed
salt and pepper to taste

Flatten chicken breasts with rolling pin. Heat 1 teaspoon oil in large skillet (or use nonstick spray). Add breasts to skillet and sauté over medium heat for 4 to 5 minutes on each side. Remove chicken from skillet. Add remaining oil, peppers, and onion. Cook vegetables until tender. Add chicken breasts, lemon juice, rosemary, salt, and pepper to vegetable mixture.

Serves 4 • Calories 210 • Carbohydrate grams 6

Tex-Mex Turkey

    4 turkey breasts (about 1 pound)
    1 teaspoon ground cumin
    salt and pepper to taste
    1 large tomato, chopped
    1 cup zucchini, chopped
    ⅓ cup sliced green onions
    1 4-ounce can diced green chili peppers, drained

Season turkey with salt, pepper, and cumin. Spray skillet with nonstick cooking spray. Cook turkey over medium heat for 10 to 12 minutes or until no longer pink, turning one time. Transfer turkey to platter. Cover with foil to keep warm. Add tomato, zucchini, onions, and chilies to skillet. Cook over high heat for 2 minutes. Spoon mixture over turkey and serve.

Serves 4 • Calories 155 • Carbohydrate grams 4

Turkey Piccata

    1 pound turkey cutlets
    1 teaspoon olive oil
    1 large clove garlic, crushed
    1 tablespoon lemon juice
    3 teaspoons capers
    salt and pepper to taste

Press turkey cutlets with garlic and pepper. Add 1 teaspoon olive oil to large skillet. Add turkey and sauté over medium heat for 4 to 5 minutes on each side. Drizzle with lemon juice and capers.

Serves 4 • Calories 230 • Carbohydrate grams 2

Turkey Roll-Ups

4   turkey breast cutlets (about 1 pound)
½   cup nonfat ricotta cheese
½   cup spinach, cooked and drained
⅛   cup bread crumbs
1½ teaspoons dried basil
½   teaspoon grated lemon peel
salt and pepper to taste
⅓   cup chicken broth
paprika

Heat oven to 350 degrees. Spray 9-inch square baking dish with nonstick cooking spray. Mix cheese, spinach, basil, bread crumbs, and lemon peel. Season turkey with salt and pepper. Spread cheese and spinach mixture over turkey. Roll breasts. Place seam-side down (or secure with toothpick). Pour broth over rolls. Sprinkle with paprika. Cover with aluminum foil. Bake 25 to 30 minutes or until turkey is done (no pink).

Serves 4 • Calories 185 • Carbohydrate grams 5

SEAFOOD

Baked Swordfish with Red Peppers and Mushrooms

4   swordfish steaks
1   cup roasted red peppers (store bought), chopped
3   cloves garlic, minced
1   tablespoon chopped parsley
½   teaspoon thyme, dried
salt and pepper to taste
1¼ cup portabello mushrooms, chopped
¼   cup dry red wine
1   tablespoon olive oil
2   tablespoons flour

Mix peppers, garlic, and thyme in small bowl. Set aside. Spray nonstick cooking spray in large ovenproof skillet. Add mushrooms. Cook over high heat for 1 minute. Add pepper mixture. Cook 1 minute. Remove and set aside.

Season swordfish steaks with salt and pepper. Lightly dust with flour. Add oil to skillet. Brown one side of steaks for 2 to 3 minutes. Turn once, browning other side for 1 to 2 minutes. Pour mushroom and pepper mixture over fish. Place skillet in oven at 350 degrees for 5 to 8 minutes or until fish is done. (Option: transfer fish into a shallow baking dish for this last step.)

Serves 4 • Calories 200 • Carbohydrate grams 4

BBQ Catfish

2   pounds catfish fillets
⅓   cup tomato sauce
½   small onion
½   clove garlic

2 tablespoons lemon juice
½ teaspoon honey
¼ teaspoon hot sauce (e.g., Tabasco)
⅛ teaspoon thyme
⅓ cup water

In large skillet, mix all ingredients except fish. Bring to boil. Reduce heat and simmer for 8 minutes. Cool sauce in refrigerator (this step can be done in advance). Spread thin layer of marinade on bottom of a glass dish. Add catfish fillets. Top fillets with marinade. Marinate for 30 minutes. Coat baking dish with nonstick cooking spray. Add fillets. Broil for 2 to 3 minutes on each side. Baste fish with reserved marinade. Fish should appear opaque when done.

Serves 4 to 5 • Calories 210 • Carbohydrate grams 3

Cioppino

8 ounces shrimp, peeled and deveined
8 ounces skinned haddock fillets, cubed
8 littleneck clams, scrubbed
1 small onion, chopped
4 green onions, sliced
2 cloves garlic, minced
1½ cups broth (chicken or vegetable)
2 cups canned tomatoes with juice, peeled and chopped (optional)
¼ cup fresh parsley, minced
1 bay leaf
⅛ teaspoon dried thyme
⅛ teaspoon dried rosemary
red and black pepper to taste

Spray large skillet with nonstick cooking spray. Add onions and garlic. Sauté over medium heat until tender. Add broth, tomatoes, parsley, bay leaf, thyme, rosemary, red pepper, and black pepper. Cover and bring to boil. Reduce heat and simmer for 30 minutes. Add shrimp, clams, and haddock. Bring to boil again. Reduce heat and simmer, covered, for 5 minutes, or until clams open, shrimp appears pink, and haddock flakes easily with fork.

Serves 4 • Calories 190 (with tomatoes and juice) •
Carbohydrate grams 10 (with tomatoes and juice)

Grilled Scallops with Portabello Mushrooms and Feta Cheese

1½ pounds scallops
½ cup fresh parsley
1½ tablespoons shallots, sliced
1 small clove garlic
½ cup dry white wine
2 tablespoons oil
4 large portabello mushrooms
1 tablespoon margarine
4 tablespoons feta cheese
1 tablespoon water

In large skillet, heat 2 tablespoons oil over medium heat. Add garlic and shallots. Cook for 1 minute. Add parsley and wine. Bring wine to boil. Add scallops. Cook for 3 to 4 minutes or until scallops appear opaque. Remove from pan. In separate baking dish, place clean portabello mushroom caps top down. Brush with margarine. Add water to dish. Dice scallops and place on mushroom caps. Bake covered for 15 to 20 minutes at

325 degrees. Remove cover and add feta cheese to mushrooms and scallops. Continue baking uncovered for 5 minutes.

Serves: 4 • Calories 180 • Carbohydrate grams 7

Grilled Swordfish with Red Pepper Salsa

- 4 swordfish steaks
- 2 tablespoons olive oil
- 1 clove garlic, pressed
- 1 to 1½ tablespoons fresh basil (½ teaspoon dried)
- 2 tablespoons lemon juice

Combine olive oil, lemon, basil, and garlic. Brush on swordfish steaks. Set aside and prepare salsa.

Salsa

- ¾ cup roasted red peppers (store bought)
- ¼ cup pitted black olives, diced
- 1 ounce Parmesan cheese
- 2 tablespoons olive oil
- 2 tablespoons chopped parsley
- 1 tablespoon fresh oregano (¼ to ½ teaspoon dried)

pepper to taste

Add ingredients together. Grill swordfish until done. To serve, spoon small amount of salsa onto each fish steak.

Salsa per ¼ cup = 100 calories, 3 carbohydrate grams

Serves 4 • Calories 200 • Carbohydrate grams 1

Halibut Brochettes

1½ pounds halibut fillets, cut into 1-inch cubes
1 tablespoon Dijon mustard
2 tablespoons olive oil
1 tablespoon lemon juice
1 tablespoon orange juice
½ teaspoon cumin
salt and pepper to taste
2 red bell peppers, cut into small pieces
wooden skewers, soaked in water for 30 minutes

In a large bowl, combine mustard, oil, cumin, orange juice, and lemon juice. Add salt and pepper to taste. Marinate halibut for at least 20 minutes. Thread red pepper pieces and halibut onto skewers. Cook over hot grill for approximately 6 to 7 minutes or until halibut is opaque.

Serves 4 • Calories 200 • Carbohydrate grams 3

Hot Shrimp

1½ pounds shrimp, cleaned
zest of 4 to 5 limes
1½ tablespoons lime juice
1 to 2 jalapeño or serrano chilies (less heat without seeds)
2 cloves garlic
2½ tablespoons chopped cilantro
1 tablespoon olive oil
wooden skewers, soaked in water for 30 minutes

Toss all ingredients together. Allow shrimp to marinate for 30 minutes. Thread shrimp onto skewers. Grill on BBQ for approximately 5 minutes, turning once. Shrimp should appear opaque.

Serves 4 • Calories 180 • Carbohydrate grams 3

Mahi-Mahi Stuffed with Veggies

1   pound mahi-mahi fillets (4)
1   large zucchini
1   small carrot
1½ tablespoons orange juice
¼   teaspoon turmeric
¼   teaspoon ginger
½   cup vegetable broth

Chop vegetables in blender. Add juice and spices. Set aside.
Spray baking dish with nonstick cooking spray. Add fish fillets.
Spread vegetable mixture over fillets. Roll fillets and secure with
toothpicks. Add broth. Bake at 325 degrees for 20 minutes or
until fish appears opaque.

Serves 4 • Calories 130 • Carbohydrate grams 4

Poached Salmon with Vegetables

4   5-ounce salmon fillets
1   cup mushrooms, quartered
1   shallot, chopped
1   clove garlic, minced
1   cup dry white wine
2   teaspoons fresh dill, chopped
2   teaspoons grated lemon peel
salt and pepper to taste
1½ cups broccoli florets
½   cup snap peas
½   teaspoon lemon juice
1   tablespoon butter

In large skillet, melt 1 teaspoon butter (or use nonstick spray).
Sauté mushrooms, shallot, and garlic for 3 minutes. Add wine

and bring to boil. Place fish in skillet. Sprinkle fillets with dill, lemon peel, salt, and pepper. Reduce heat, cover, and simmer for 3 minutes. Add broccoli and snap peas. Simmer for additional 2 minutes. Fish should appear opaque and flake easily with a fork. Remove fish. Add lemon and butter (optional) to pan juices. Serve over fish.

Serves 4 • Calories 300 • Carbohydrate grams 4
(calorie and gram amounts include vegetables)

Poached Sole with Italian Vegetables

4   5-ounce sole fillets
1   cup chicken broth or vegetable stock
1   medium tomato, peeled and chopped
1   green pepper, cut into thin strips
1   small onion, diced
1   clove garlic, minced
2   tablespoons Parmesan cheese

Add broth, tomato, green pepper, onion, and garlic to large skillet. Bring to boil. Add fillets. Reduce heat and simmer, covered, for 4 to 6 minutes. Fish should appear opaque and flake easily with a fork.

Serves 4 • Calories 170 • Carbohydrate grams 4

Red Snapper Victoria

1½ pounds snapper fillets
1   clove garlic, pressed
2   tablespoons olive oil
1   15-ounce can tomato sauce (optional)
2   stalks celery, sliced
1   medium carrot, sliced thin

1 16-ounce can stewed tomatoes (optional)
1 medium onion, chopped
1 teaspoon oregano
1 teaspoon basil
1 teaspoon garlic salt
pepper to taste

Add oil to large skillet. Sauté garlic. Add onion, celery, and carrots. Sauté until celery appears translucent. Add tomato sauce,
chopped tomatoes, and herbs. Bring to boil. Reduce heat and
simmer, covered, for 10 minutes. Add red snapper fillets. Bring to
boil again. Reduce heat and simmer for 15 minutes or until fish
flakes easily with a fork.

> Serves 4 • Calories 280 (with tomatoes and sauce) •
> Calories 240 (without tomatoes and sauce) •
> Carbohydrate grams 12 (with tomatoes and sauce) •
> Carbohydrate grams 3 (without tomatoes and sauce)

Salmon with Cabernet Sauce

4 salmon fillets
1½ cups Cabernet wine
¼ cup tarragon vinegar
¼ cup shallots, minced
4 sprigs fresh tarragon
parsley (for garnish)
1 teaspoon whole black peppercorns

Spray nonstick cooking spray onto large baking dish. Arrange
salmon fillets in dish. Top each fillet with 1 sprig tarragon. Bake
at 400 degrees for 10 minutes or until fish is opaque and flakes
easily with a fork.

Combine remaining ingredients in saucepan. Bring sauce to a boil. Reduce heat and simmer. Spoon over fish. (Optional: Whisk ½ stick butter into sauce while boiling.)

Serves 4 • Calories 270 (sauce without butter) •
Calories 370 (sauce with butter) • Carbohydrate grams 4

Salmon Fillet with Dill and Leeks en Papillotte

4   salmon fillets
½   cup dry white wine
½   cup leeks, chopped
2   tablespoons fresh dill, chopped
1   tablespoon green pepper sauce (store bought)
1   tablespoon lime juice
salt to taste

Combine wine, leeks, dill, pepper sauce, lime juice, and salt in small bowl. Place salmon fillets on individual pieces of foil or parchment paper. Pour wine mixture over each fillet. Close foil or paper over fish, sealing edges. Place on baking pan. Bake at 375 degrees for 20 to 25 minutes or until fish flakes easily with a fork.

Serves 4 • Calories 290 • Carbohydrate grams 2

Scallop Ceviche

1   pound bay scallops, cleaned
1   bay leaf
4   scallions, chopped, white part only
⅓   cup grapefruit juice
¼   cup lime juice
1   tablespoon lime zest

1   tablespoon grapefruit zest
4   tablespoons olive oil
¼   cup red onion, chopped
¼   cup red bell pepper, chopped
1 to 2 tablespoons cilantro, chopped
1   teaspoon oregano, dried
salt and pepper to taste

In large pot, bring water to a boil. Add bay leaf to water. Add cleaned scallops and boil for 3 minutes. Remove scallops and immediately place in ice water (this will firm the scallops).

    In small bowl, mix remaining ingredients. Cut or tear scallops into small pieces. Mix with marinade and chill. Serve in lettuce cups.

Serves 4 • Calories 220 • Carbohydrate grams 7

Shrimp Mediterranean

1   pound shrimp, peeled and deveined
2   tablespoons olive oil
1   small red onion
2   cups Italian plum tomatoes, drained and chopped
½   cup dry white wine
1 to 1½ teaspoons dried oregano
salt and pepper to taste
2   ounces feta cheese

Heat oil in large skillet over medium heat. Sauté onion until translucent. Add tomatoes, wine, and oregano. Reduce heat and simmer until sauce thickens, about 5 minutes. Add shrimp. Stir and cook until shrimp appears opaque, about 3 minutes. Add salt and pepper to taste. Sprinkle with feta cheese.

Serves 4 • Calories 260 (with tomatoes) •
Calories 220 (without tomatoes) •
Carbohydrate grams 12 (with tomatoes) •
Carbohydrate grams 3 (without tomatoes) •

Sole with Mustard and Dill

4   7-ounce sole fillets
¼   cup lemon juice
3 to 4 tablespoons Dijon mustard
1   teaspoon dried dill

Spray broiler pan with nonstick cooking spray. Add fillets. Pour lemon juice over fillets. Fold in half and secure with toothpicks. Mix remaining ingredients. Spoon over fillets. Place pan on top rack of oven. Cook 7 to 10 minutes or until fish is opaque and flakes easily.

Serves 4 • Calories 175 • Carbohydrate grams 2

Spinach-Stuffed Flounder with Mushrooms and Feta Cheese

4   5-ounce flounder fillets (option: orange roughy or sole)
nonstick cooking spray
8   large mushrooms, thinly sliced
8   ounces spinach, chopped
1   tablespoon feta cheese
2   tablespoons water

Spray large skillet with nonstick cooking spray. Add mushrooms and spinach. Sauté until spinach is slightly wilted. Drain off any liquid. Add feta. Set aside. Spray large baking dish with nonstick cooking spray. Add fillets. Place spinach, mushroom, and feta mixture on each fillet. Roll fillets and secure with toothpicks. Add 2 tablespoons water to dish. Cover with foil and bake at 350 degrees for 15 to 20 minutes. Fish should appear opaque and flake easily with a fork.

Serves 4 • Calories 150 • Carbohydrate grams 2

Swordfish in Chardonnay Sauce

4   swordfish steaks (option: salmon or mahi-mahi)
1   cup Chardonnay wine
¼   cup lemon juice
1 to 2 tablespoons lemon zest
1   teaspoon vanilla extract
⅛   cup olive oil
1   teaspoon diced jalapeño pepper (without seeds)
2   garlic cloves, crushed
salt to taste

Whisk Chardonnay, lemon juice, zest, and vanilla together in small bowl. Add oil slowly while whisking. Add jalapeño, garlic, and salt. Marinate fish for 45 minutes to 1 hour.

Place swordfish steaks on hot grill. Cook for 5 minutes. Turn once and grill for 4 minutes or until fish is opaque.

Serves 4 • Calories 230 • Carbohydrate grams 2

Swordfish Kebabs

2 pounds swordfish
¼ cup canola oil
⅓ cup lemon juice
1 tablespoon crushed garlic
1 tablespoon gingerroot, minced (1 to 1½ teaspoons powdered ginger)
1 bay leaf, crumbled
salt to taste
wooden skewers, soaked in water for 30 minutes

Cube swordfish into 1- to ½-inch pieces. Thread pieces onto skewers. Whisk remaining ingredients together. Brush over kebabs. Grill over high heat for 6 to 8 minutes, turning often and basting with marinade.

Serves 4 • Calories 250 • Carbohydrate grams 2

Tamari Mahi-Mahi

4 7-ounce mahi-mahi fillets
1¾ teaspoons sesame oil
1 tablespoon tamari sauce
1 tablespoon mirin
1 tablespoon rice vinegar (unsweetened)
2 scallions, thinly sliced
pepper to taste

Mix 1 teaspoon oil with tamari, mirin, and vinegar. Add remaining oil to skillet. Over medium heat, lightly brown fish on bottom for 1 to 2 minutes. Turn fish once and reduce heat to low. Add sauce and cover. Steam mahi-mahi over low heat for 4 to 5 minutes. Turn and cook for 2 to 3 minutes. Fish should be opaque.

Remove fish from skillet. Add scallions to pan juices. Allow sauce to reduce. Spoon over fish.

Serves 4 • Calories 140 • Carbohydrate grams 2

Tuna with Lemon and Sorrel

4 large tuna steaks
½ teaspoon brown mustard
⅛ cup lemon juice
2 tablespoons balsamic vinegar
3 tablespoons olive oil
½ teaspoon thyme, dried
3 tablespoons sorrel leaves
salt and pepper to taste

In small bowl, mix mustard, lemon juice, vinegar, 2 tablespoons olive oil, thyme, and sorrel. Place tuna steaks in large dish. Cover with marinade. Marinate for at least 1 hour (preferably 2 to 3 hours). Add 1 tablespoon oil to large skillet. Heat on high until oil begins to smoke. Add steaks. Sear on one side for 3 to 4 minutes until brown. Turn and sear on other side for 3 minutes.

Serves 4 • Calories 200 • Carbohydrate grams 2

BEEF AND PORK

Beef Brisket with Chipotle Pepper Rub

2½ pounds brisket

1 tablespoon lime juice

2 tablespoons dry red wine

3 tablespoons olive oil

1 tablespoon cracked black pepper

2 tablespoons dried oregano

1 teaspoon cumin

1½ teaspoons onion powder

3 dried chipotle peppers, crushed (remove seeds for less heat)

1 tablespoon dried cilantro

Grind all dry ingredients into a powder. Add oil, wine, and lime juice. Coat brisket. Marinate overnight or up to three days. To cook, heat oven to 200 degrees. Roast brisket for 2 hours per pound. Start this one in the morning!

Makes 10 to 12 4-ounce servings • Calories 275 •
Carbohydrate grams 1

Beef Rolls

1 pound round, thinly sliced into 8 strips

¼ cup sesame oil

5 cloves garlic, pressed

3 tablespoons shallots, chopped

3 tablespoons gingerroot, finely chopped

1 tablespoon sherry vinegar

8   large scallions
¼   cup sake
½   cup soy sauce

In a large bowl, combine sesame oil, soy sauce, garlic, shallots, gingerroot, vinegar, and sake. Add thin strips of beef and shallots and marinate for at least 30 minutes. Place strips on baking dish. Place 1 scallion on each piece of beef. Roll each slice of beef and secure with toothpick. Broil for 6 to 7 minutes or until desired doneness.

Serves 4 • Calories 250 • Carbohydrate grams 2

Rosemary Pork Brochettes

1½ pounds pork loin, cut into 1-inch cubes
2   tablespoons olive oil
¼   cup red wine vinegar
1   tablespoon rosemary
1   small clove garlic, finely chopped
1   teaspoon cumin
salt and pepper to taste
red pepper flakes to taste
wooden skewers, soaked in water for 30 minutes

Mix 1 tablespoon oil, vinegar, rosemary, garlic, cumin, salt, and pepper (red or black) in large bowl. Add pork. Marinate for at least 40 minutes. Thread pork onto skewers. Place on hot grill. Use remaining oil on grill as needed. Turn brochettes often for 17 to 20 minutes or until pork is done.

Serves 4 • Calories 320 • Carbohydrate grams 1

Beef Satay

1 pound top round, trimmed and cut into small strips
1 tablespoon sesame oil
4 tablespoons soy sauce
2 tablespoons rice vinegar, unsweetened
1 tablespoon brown sugar
1 clove garlic, minced
1 teaspoon red pepper flakes
wooden skewers, soaked in water for 30 minutes

In a large bowl, combine soy sauce, sesame oil, sugar, vinegar, garlic, and pepper. Combine beef with mixture. Marinate beef for at least 30 minutes. Thread beef onto skewers. Grill for 2 to 3 minutes on each side or until beef is done.

Serves 4 • Calories 250 • Carbohydrate grams 3

Grilled Flank Steak

1 pound flank steak
2 tablespoons olive oil
2 tablespoons fresh lemon juice
2 tablespoons dry red wine
2 teaspoons dried basil
3 large shallots, chopped

Mix olive oil, wine, lemon juice, thyme, basil, and shallots in small bowl. Place flank steak in large glass dish. Cover with marinade. Marinate steak for at least 30 minutes. Place steak on hot grill. Grill until desired doneness. Cut against grain into thin strips.

Serves 4 • Calories 240 • Carbohydrate grams 1

Island Pork Loin

4   pork loin steaks
3   cloves garlic, diced
1   small onion, finely chopped
2   celery stalks, finely chopped
2 to 3 jalapeño peppers, diced (remove seeds for less heat)
1   tablespoon thyme
¼   cup lime juice
salt and pepper to taste

Combine garlic, onion, celery, lime juice, diced peppers, and thyme in food processor. Blend until finely minced together. Add salt and pepper. Place mixture on pork loin steaks and marinate for at least 40 minutes. Broil on top rack for 10 minutes on each side.

Serves 4 • Calories 320 • Carbohydrate grams 6

Spanish Pork Loin

4   pork loin steaks
2   tablespoons olive oil
1   large clove garlic, mashed
1   tablespoon paprika
½   teaspoon oregano
2   tablespoons lemon juice
1   bay leaf, crumbled
salt and pepper to taste

Mix oil, garlic, oregano, paprika, bay leaf, and lemon juice together. Pour over steaks. Marinate pork loin steaks for at least 40 minutes. Broil on top rack for 10 minutes on each side.

Serves 4 • Calories 250 • Carbohydrate grams 2

Wine and Herb Beef

1 pound flank steak (optional: other cuts if preferred)
⅛ cup sherry vinegar (or red wine vinegar)
¼ cup dry red wine
2 tablespoons soy sauce
½ teaspoon Worcestershire sauce
½ teaspoon sugar
⅛ cup olive oil
1 large clove garlic, crushed
1 tablespoon parsley
½ teaspoon dried rosemary
½ teaspoon dried tarragon
½ teaspoon dried thyme
black pepper to taste

Mix all ingredients in small bowl. Place flank steak in large dish. Cover with marinade. Marinate for at least 30 minutes. Place steak on hot grill. Use reserved marinade for basting. Cook until desired doneness.

Serves 4 • Calories 250 • Carbohydrate grams 3

TOFU

Curry Seasoned Tofu

16 ounces firm tofu, cut into 1-inch cubes
2 tablespoons curry powder
½ teaspoon cinnamon
2 dried red chilies, crumbled (remove seeds for less heat)
1 tablespoon sherry
2 tablespoons lemon juice

2   tablespoons lime juice
2   tablespoons peanut oil (substitute canola or safflower
    if desired)
1   tablespoon shallots, finely chopped
cilantro, to taste

Mix all ingredients in large bowl. Add tofu cubes. Marinate for at
least 30 minutes. Add 1 tablespoon oil to large skillet. Add tofu.
Cook over medium-high heat for 4 minutes or until cooked
on all sides.

Serves 4 • Calories 230 • Carbohydrate grams 6

Tofu and Portabello Stir-Fry

16 ounces firm tofu, cut into 1-inch cubes
2   large portabello mushroom caps, chopped
1   red bell pepper, cut into 1-inch strips
1   small onion, cut into small strips
¼   pound bean sprouts
1   bunch bok choy
2 to 3 chipotle peppers, crumbled
2   cloves garlic, finely minced
2 to 3 tablespoons sesame oil (canola or safflower if desired)
soy sauce to taste

Place portabello mushrooms and tofu in two separate bowls.
Cover with desired amount of soy sauce. Heat large wok or skillet
on low heat. Add oil and garlic. Cook uncovered until slightly
browned. Add peppers. Cook 1 minute. Add tofu. Cook
uncovered for 10 minutes. Add mushrooms and cook for an
additional 3 minutes. Add remaining vegetables and cook
covered for 3 to 5 minutes.

Serves 4 • Calories 250 • Carbohydrate grams 11

Tofu and Mixed Vegetable Stir-Fry

16 ounces tofu, cut into 1-inch cubes
¼ cup soy sauce
¼ cup rice vinegar, unsweetened
2 teaspoons powdered ginger
2 small cloves garlic, minced
2 medium Chinese eggplants, chopped
½ pound shiitake mushrooms, chopped
small bunch broccoli, cut into small pieces
3 tablespoons scallions, chopped
2 tablespoons sesame oil
½ packet sweetener
hot sauce to taste

In small bowl, mix soy sauce, vinegar, sweetener, desired amount of hot sauce, and tofu. Set aside. Heat oil in large wok or skillet over medium-high heat. Add garlic and ginger. Cook until garlic is slightly browned. Add tofu. Cook uncovered for 10 minutes. Add remaining ingredients. Cover and cook for 5 minutes.

Serves 4 • Calories 250 • Carbohydrate grams 10

Tofu with Three Cheeses

10 ounces tofu, sliced
1 cup ricotta cheese
¼ cup Parmesan cheese
1 large egg white
¼ teaspoon ground nutmeg
¼ teaspoon white pepper
1 small clove garlic, minced
⅓ cup tomato sauce
2 small Roma tomatoes, sliced

½ cup basil, chopped
1 cup shredded nonfat mozzarella cheese

Mix ricotta cheese, Parmesan cheese, egg white, 2 to 3 table-spoons tomato sauce, garlic, nutmeg, and pepper in small bowl. Add ¼ cup tomato sauce to 8-inch square baking dish. Cut tofu into thin slices. Place layer of tofu in dish. Layer with cheese mix-ture. Layer with tomato, followed by basil and mozzarella cheese. Bake at 350 degrees for 15 to 20 minutes or until cheese is melted and slightly bubbling.

Serves 4 • Calories 225 • Carbohydrate grams 6

Food Composition Tables*

Name	Amount	Calories	Carbohydrate (g)	Protein (g)	Fat (g)
Beverages					
beer, regular	12 fl oz	150	13	1	0
beer, light	12 fl oz	95	5	1	0
gin, rum, vodka,					
whiskey, 80-proof	1.5 fl oz	95	0	0	0
wine, dessert	3.5 fl oz	140	8	0	0

*Food categories are listed in alphabetical order. For example, "blueberries" are listed under "fruit." Food categories are as follows: beverages; cheese; dairy products; dressings; eggs; fats, fish and shellfish; fruit; grains/starches, meat; meat products; meals/prepared recipes; nuts and seeds; poultry; sauces; soups; soy foods; sweets; vegetables; and miscellaneous items.

Reading nutrient columns: Nutrients are listed from left to right in the following order: calories, carbohydrate grams, protein grams, fat grams.

Source: USDA Department of Agriculture, Agricultural Research Service, 1998. USDA Nutrient Database for Standard Reference, release 12. Nutrient data laboratory home page: http://www.nal.usda.gov/fnic/foodcomp

Name	Amount	Calories	Carbohydrate (g)	Protein (g)	Fat (g)
wine, table, red	3.5 fl oz	75	3	0	0
wine, table, white	3.5 fl oz	80	3	0	0
club soda	12 fl oz	0	0	0	0
cola, regular	12 fl oz	160	41	0	0
cola, diet,					
aspartame/saccharin	12 fl oz	0	0	0	0
ginger ale	12 fl oz	125	32	0	0
grape soda	12 fl oz	180	46	0	0
lemon-lime soda	12 fl oz	155	39	0	0
orange soda	12 fl oz	180	46	0	0
root beer	12 fl oz	165	42	0	0
coffee, brewed	4 fl oz	0	0	0	0
coffee, instant, prepared	4 fl oz	0	1	0	0
fruit punch drink, canned	4 fl oz	57	14	0	0
grape drink, canned	4 fl oz	68	17	0	0
lemonade, concentrated, frozen,					
diluted	4 fl oz	56	14	0	0
tea, brewed	4 fl oz	0	0	0	0

Name	Amount	Calories	Carbohydrate (g)	Protein (g)	Fat (g)
tea, instant, prepared					
unsweetened	4 fl oz	0	0	0	0
sweetened	4 fl oz	44	11	0	0
Cheese					
blue cheese	1 oz	100	1	6	8
Camembert cheese	1 wedge	115	0	8	9
cheddar cheese	1 oz	115	0	7	9
cheddar cheese, shredded	1 cup	455	1	28	37
cottage cheese, creamed, small curd	1 cup	215	6	26	9
cottage cheese, creamed, w/fruit	1 cup	280	30	22	8
cottage cheese, lowfat 2%	1 cup	205	8	31	4
cream cheese	1 oz	100	1	2	10
feta cheese	1 oz	75	1	4	6
mozzarella cheese, skim, low moisture	1 oz	80	1	8	5

Name	Amount	Calories	Carbohydrate (g)	Protein (g)	Fat (g)
Muenster cheese	1 oz	105	0	7	9
Parmesan cheese, grated	1 oz	130	1	12	9
Parmesan cheese, grated	1 tbsp	25	0	2	2
provolone cheese	1 oz	100	1	7	8
ricotta cheese, whole milk	1 cup	430	7	28	32
ricotta cheese, part skim milk	1 cup	340	13	28	19
ricotta cheese, part skim milk	1 oz	85	3	7	5
Swiss cheese	1 oz	105	1	8	8
pasteurized processed cheese					
American	1 oz	105	0	6	9
Swiss	1 oz	95	1	7	7
cheese food (American)	1 oz	95	2	6	7
cheese spread (American)	1 oz	80	2	5	6
Dairy Products					
cream, half and half	1 tbsp	20	1	0	2
coffee or table cream, light	1 tbsp	30	1	0	3
whipping cream, unwhipped, light	1 tbsp	45	0	0	5

Name	Amount	Calories	Carbohydrate (g)	Protein (g)	Fat (g)
whipped topping, pressurized	½ cup	78	4	1	6
whipped topping, pressurized	1 tbsp	10	0	0	1
sour cream	1 tbsp	25	1	0	3
imitation whipped topping, pressurized	1 tbsp	10	1	0	1
imitation sour cream dressing	1 tbsp	20	1	0	2
milk					
lowfat, 2%, no added solids	1 cup	120	12	8	5
lowfat, 1%, no added solids	1 cup	100	12	8	3
skim, no added solids	1 cup	85	12	8	0
buttermilk, fluid	1 cup	100	12	8	2
evaporated milk, skim, canned	1 cup	200	29	19	1
buttermilk, dried	1 cup	465	59	41	7
nonfat dry milk, instant	1 cup	245	35	24	0
chocolate milk, regular	1 cup	210	26	8	8
eggnog	1 cup	340	34	10	19
ice cream, vanilla, regular, 11% fat	1 cup	270	32	5	14
ice cream, vanilla, soft serve	1 cup	375	38	7	23

Name	Amount	Calories	Carbohydrate (g)	Protein (g)	Fat (g)
ice cream, vanilla, rich, 16% fat	1 cup	350	32	4	24
ice milk, vanilla, soft serve 3% fat	1 cup	225	38	8	5
sherbet, 2% fat	1 cup	270	59	2	4
yogurt, w/low fat milk, fruit flavored	1 cup	230	43	10	2
yogurt, w/low fat milk, plain	1	145	16	12	4
yogurt, w/nonfat milk	1	125	17	13	0
Dressings					
blue cheese salad dressing	1 tbsp	75	1	1	8
French salad dressing, regular	1 tbsp	85	1	0	9
French salad dressing, lowcal	1 tbsp	25	2	0	2
Italian salad dressing, regular	1 tbsp	80	1	0	9
Italian salad dressing, lowcal	1 tbsp	5	2	0	0
mayonnaise, regular	1 tbsp	100	0	0	11
mayonnaise, imitation	1 tbsp	35	2	0	3
mayonnaise-type salad dressing	1 tbsp	60	4	0	5
tartar sauce	1 tbsp	75	1	0	8
1000 Island dressing, regular	1 tbsp	60	2	0	6

Name	Amount	Calories	Carbohydrate (g)	Protein (g)	Fat (g)
1000 Island dressing, lowcal	1 tbsp	25	2	0	2
vinegar and oil salad dressing	1 tbsp	70	0	0	8
Eggs					
eggs, raw, whole	1	75	1	6	5
eggs, raw, white	1	15	0	4	0
Fats					
butter, salted	1 tbsp	100	0	0	11
butter, unsalted	1 tbsp	100	0	0	11
vegetable shortening	1 tbsp	115	0	0	13
lard	1 tbsp	115	0	0	13
margarine, regular					
hard, 80% fat	1 tbsp	35	0	0	4
soft, 80% fat	1 tbsp	75	0	0	9
corn oil	1 tbsp	125	0	0	14
olive oil	1 tbsp	125	0	0	14
peanut oil	1 tbsp	125	0	0	14
safflower oil	1 tbsp	125	0	0	14

Name	Amount	Calories	Carbohydrate (g)	Protein (g)	Fat (g)
soybean oil, hydrogenated	1 tbsp	125	0	0	14
soybean/cottonseed oil, hydrogenated	1 tbsp	125	0	0	14
sunflower oil	1 tbsp	125	0	0	14
Fish and Shellfish					
clams, raw	3 oz	65	2	11	1
clams, canned, drained	3 oz	85	2	13	2
crabmeat, canned	1 cup	135	1	23	3
crabmeat, steamed	3 oz	80	0	15	2
fish sticks, frozen, reheated	1 stick	70	4	6	3
flounder or sole, baked, butter	3 oz	120	0	16	6
flounder or sole, baked, no fat	3 oz	80	0	17	1
haddock, breaded, fried	3 oz	175	7	17	9
halibut, broiled, butter, lemon juice	3	140	0	20	6
halibut, Atlantic/Pacific, meat only, raw	3 oz	114	0	24	2
herring, pickled	3 oz	190	0	17	13

Name	Amount	Calories	Carbohydrate (g)	Protein (g)	Fat (g)
oysters, raw	1 cup	160	8	20	4
oysters, breaded, fried	1	90	5	5	5
salmon, canned, pink, w/bones	3 oz	120	0	17	5
salmon, baked, red	3 oz	140	0	21	5
salmon, smoked	3 oz	150	0	18	8
sardines, Atlantic, canned in oil, drained	3 oz	175	0	20	9
sea bass, white, flesh only, raw	3 oz	82	0	18	1
scallops, raw	3 oz	69	3	13	0
shrimp, canned, drained	3 oz	100	1	21	1
shrimp, French fried	3 oz	200	11	16	10
trout, broiled, w/butter, lemon juice	3 oz	175	0	21	9
trout, brook, flesh only	3 oz	86	0	16	2
tuna, canned, drained, oil chunk light	3 oz	165	0	24	7
tuna, canned, drained, water, white	3 oz	135	0	30	1
tuna salad	1 cup	375	19	33	19

Name	Amount	Calories	Carbohydrate (g)	Protein (g)	Fat (g)
Fruit					
apples, raw, unpeeled, 3 per lb	1	80	21	0	0
apples, raw, peeled, sliced	1 cup	65	16	0	0
apples, dried, sulfured	10 rings	155	42	1	0
apple juice, canned	1 cup	115	29	0	0
applesauce, canned, unsweetened	1 cup	105	28	0	0
apricots, raw	3	50	12	1	0
apricots, canned, heavy syrup	3 halves	70	18	0	0
apricots, canned, juice pack	1 cup	120	31	2	0
apricots, canned, juice pack	3 halves	40	10	1	0
apricots, dried, cooked, unsweetened	1 cup	210	55	3	0
apricot nectar, no added vitamin C	1 cup	140	36	1	0
avocados, California	1	305	12	4	30
avocados, Florida	1	340	27	5	27
bananas	1	105	27	1	1
bananas, sliced	1 cup	140	35	2	1
blackberries, raw	1 cup	75	18	1	1

Name	Amount	Calories	Carbohydrate (g)	Protein (g)	Fat (g)
blueberries, raw	1 cup	80	20	1	1
blueberries, frozen, sweetened	1 cup	185	50	1	0
cherries, sour, red, canned, water	1 cup	90	22	2	0
cherries, sweet, raw	10	50	11	1	1
cranberry juice cocktail w/vitamin C	1 cup	145	38	0	0
cranberry sauce, canned, sweetened	1 cup	420	108	1	0
dates	10	230	61	2	0
figs, dried	10	475	122	6	2
fruit cocktail, canned, juice pack	1 cup	115	29	1	0
grapefruit, raw, pink, white	½	40	10	1	0
grapefruit, canned, syrup pack	1 cup	150	39	1	0
grapefruit juice, raw	1 cup	95	23	1	0
grapes, European, raw, Thompson	10	35	9	0	0
grape juice, canned	1 cup	155	38	1	0
grape juice, frozen, diluted, sweetened, w/vitamin C	1 cup	125	32	0	0
kiwi fruit, raw	1	45	11	1	0

Name	Amount	Calories	Carbohydrate (g)	Protein (g)	Fat (g)
lemons/limes, raw	1	15	5	1	0
lemon/lime juice, canned	1 tbsp	5	1	0	0
mangos, raw	1	135	35	1	1
cantaloupe, raw	½	95	22	2	1
honeydew melon, raw	⅒	45	12	1	0
nectarines, raw	1	65	16	1	1
oranges, raw	1	60	15	1	0
orange juice, chilled	1 cup	110	25	2	1
papayas, raw	1 cup	65	17	1	0
peaches, raw	1	35	10	1	0
peaches, canned, juice pack	1 cup	110	29	2	0
pears, raw, Bartlett	1	100	25	1	1
pears, canned, juice pack	1 cup	125	32	1	0
pineapple, raw, diced	1 cup	75	19	1	1
pineapple, canned, juice pack	1 cup	150	39	1	0
plums, raw, 2⅛ inch	1	35	9	1	0
plums, canned, juice pack	3	55	14	0	0

Name	Amount	Calories	Carbohydrate (g)	Protein (g)	Fat (g)
prunes, dried	5 large	115	31	1	0
prunes, dried, cooked, unsweetened	1 cup	225	60	2	0
prune juice, canned	1 cup	180	45	2	0
raisins	1 cup	435	115	5	1
raisins	1 packet	40	11	0	0
raspberries, raw	1 cup	60	14	1	1
rhubarb, cooked, sugar added	1 cup	280	75	1	0
strawberries, raw	1 cup	45	10	1	1
strawberries, frozen, sweetened	1 cup	245	66	1	0
tangerines, raw	1	35	9	1	0
watermelon, raw	1 piece	155	35	3	2
watermelon, raw, diced	1 cup	50	11	1	1

Grains/Starches

Breads, cereals, cakes, pasta, rice, etc.

Name	Amount	Calories	Carbohydrate (g)	Protein (g)	Fat (g)
bagels, plain	1	200	38	7	2
baking powder biscuits, from mix	1	95	14	2	3

Name	Amount	Calories	Carbohydrate (g)	Protein (g)	Fat (g)
bread crumbs, dry, grated	1 cup	390	73	13	5
cracked-wheat bread	1 slice	65	12	2	1
French bread	1 slice	100	18	3	1
Vienna bread	1 slice	70	13	2	1
Italian bread	1 slice	85	17	3	0
mixed-grain bread	1 slice	65	12	2	1
oatmeal bread	1 slice	65	12	2	1
pita bread	1	165	33	6	1
pumpernickel bread	1 slice	80	16	3	1
raisin bread	1 slice	65	13	2	1
rye bread, light	1 slice	65	12	2	1
wheat bread	1 slice	65	12	2	1
wheat bread, toasted	1 slice	65	12	3	1
whole-wheat bread	1 slice	70	13	3	1
bread stuffing, from mix, moist	1 cup	420	40	9	26
corn grits, cracked, regular, yellow, no salt	1 cup	145	31	3	0
cream of wheat, instant, no salt	1 cup	140	29	4	0

Name	Amount	Calories	Carbohydrate (g)	Protein (g)	Fat (g)
Malt-o-Meal, w/o salt (cooked)	1 cup	120	26	4	0
oatmeal (cooked)					
regular instant (no salt)	1 cup	145	25	6	2
instant, plain, fortified	1 packet	105	18	4	2
All-Bran cereal	1 oz	70	21	4	1
Cheerios cereal	1 oz	110	20	4	2
corn flakes, Kellogg's	1 oz	110	24	2	0
40% bran flakes, Post	1 oz	90	22	3	0
Golden Grahams cereal	1 oz	110	24	2	1
Grape-Nuts cereal	1 oz	100	23	3	0
Nature Valley Granola cereal	1 oz	125	19	3	5
Product 19 cereal	1 oz	110	24	3	0
raisin bran, Post	1 oz	85	21	3	1
Rice Krispies cereal	1 oz	110	25	2	0
Shredded wheat cereal	1 oz	100	23	3	1
Special K cereal	1 oz	110	21	6	0
Total cereal	1 oz	100	22	3	1

Name	Amount	Calories	Carbohydrate (g)	Protein (g)	Fat (g)
Wheaties cereal	1 oz	100	23	3	0
buckwheat flour, light, sifted	1 cup	340	78	6	1
angel food cake, from mix	1 piece	125	29	3	0
coffeecake, crumb, from mix	1 piece	230	38	5	7
devil's food cake, chocolate frosting, from mix	1 piece	235	40	3	8
devil's food cake, chocolate frosting, from mix	1 cupcake	120	20	2	4
gingerbread cake, from mix	1 piece	175	32	2	4
yellow cake, chocolate frosting, from mix	1 piece	235	40	3	8
carrot cake, cream cheese frosting, homemade	1 piece	385	48	4	21
fruitcake, dark, homemade	1 piece	165	25	2	7
sheet cake, white frosting, homemade	1 piece	445	77	4	14
pound cake, homemade	1 loaf	2,025	265	33	94
pound cake, homemade	1 slice	120	15	2	5

Name	Amount	Calories	Carbohydrate (g)	Protein (g)	Fat (g)
pound cake, bakery	1 slice	110	15	2	5
white cake, white frosting, bakery	1 piece	260	42	3	9
yellow cake, chocolate frosting, bakery	1 piece	245	39	2	11
cheesecake	1 piece	280	26	5	18
brownie w/nuts, frosting, bakery	1	100	16	1	4
chocolate chip cookies,bakery	4	180	28	2	9
chocolate chip cookies, slice and bake	4	225	32	2	11
fig bars	4	210	42	2	4
oatmeal and raisin cookie	4	245	36	3	10
peanut butter cookie,homemade	4	245	28	4	14
sandwich-type cookie	4	195	29	2	8
sugar cookie, slice and bake	4	235	31	2	12
corn chips	1 oz	155	16	2	9
cornmeal, degermed, enriched	1 cup	120	26	3	0
cheese crackers, plain	10	50	6	1	3
cheese-and-peanut-butter-sandwich crackers	1	40	5	1	2

Name	Amount	Calories	Carbohydrate (g)	Protein (g)	Fat (g)
Graham cracker, plain	2	60	11	1	1
melba toast, plain	1 piece	20	4	1	0
rye wafers, whole grain	2	55	10	1	1
saltines	4	50	9	1	1
snack-type crackers	1	15	2	0	1
thin wheat crackers	4	35	5	1	1
whole-wheat wafers, crackers	2	35	5	1	2
croissants	1	235	27	5	12
Danish pastry, plain, no nuts	1	220	26	4	12
Danish pastry, plain, no nuts	1 oz	110	13	2	6
Danish pastry, fruit	1	235	28	4	13
doughnuts, cake type, plain	1	210	24	3	12
doughnuts, yeast-leavened, glazed	1	235	26	4	13
English muffin, plain	1	140	27	5	1
French toast, home recipe	1 slice	155	17	6	7
macaroni, cooked	1 cup	155	32	5	1
blueberry muffins, from mix	1	140	22	3	5
bran muffins, from mix	1	140	24	3	4

Name	Amount	Calories	Carbohydrate (g)	Protein (g)	Fat (g)
corn muffins, from mix	1	145	22	3	6
noodles, egg, cooked	1 cup	200	37	7	2
noodles, chow mein, canned	1 cup	220	26	6	11
pancakes, plain, from mix	1	60	8	2	2
apple pie	1 piece	405	60	3	18
blueberry pie	1 piece	380	55	4	17
cherry pie	1 piece	410	61	4	18
cream pie	1 piece	455	59	3	23
pecan pie	1 piece	575	71	7	32
pumpkin pie	1 piece	320	37	6	17
popcorn, air-popped, unsalted	1 cup	30	6	1	0
popcorn, popped, in vegetable oil, salted	1 cup	55	6	1	3
pretzels, stick	10	10	2	0	0
rice, brown, cooked	1 cup	230	50	5	1
rice, white, cooked	1 cup	225	50	4	0
rolls, dinner, bakery	1	85	14	2	2
rolls, frankfurter, hamburger	1	115	20	3	2

Name	Amount	Calories	Carbohydrate (g)	Protein (g)	Fat (g)
rolls, hard	1	155	30	5	2
rolls, hoagie or submarine	1	400	72	11	8
spaghetti, cooked	1 cup	155	32	5	1
tortillas, corn	1	65	13	2	1
waffles, from mix	1	205	27	7	8
wheat flour, all-purpose, sifted	1 cup	420	88	12	1
Beans, peas, legumes					
black beans, dry, cooked, drained	1 cup	225	41	15	1
lentils, dry, cooked	1 cup	180	4	4	18
lima beans, baby, frozen, cooked	1 cup	190	35	12	1
pea beans, dry, cooked	1 cup	225	40	15	1
pinto beans, dry, cooked	1 cup	265	49	15	1
red kidney beans, dry, canned	1 cup	230	42	15	1
black-eyed peas, dry, cooked	1 cup	190	35	13	1
peas, split, dry, cooked	1 cup	230	42	16	1

Name	Amount	Calories	Carbohydrate (g)	Protein (g)	Fat (g)
Meat					
Beef					
cooked, chuck blade, lean and fat	3 oz	325	0	22	26
cooked, bottom round, lean and fat	3 oz	220	0	25	13
cooked, bottom round, lean only	2.8 oz	175	0	25	8
ground beef, broiled, lean	3 oz	230	0	21	16
ground beef, broiled, regular	3 oz	245	0	20	18
beef roast, rib, lean and fat	3 oz	315	0	19	26
beef roast, rib, lean only	2.2 oz	150	0	17	9
beef roast, round eye, lean and fat	3 oz	205	0	23	12
beef roast, round eye, lean only	2.6 oz	135	0	22	5
beef steak, sirloin, broiled, lean and fat	3 oz	240	0	23	15
beef steak, sirloin, broiled, lean only	2.5 oz	150	0	22	6
beef, canned, corned	3 oz	185	0	22	10

Name	Amount	Calories	Carbohydrate (g)	Protein (g)	Fat (g)
lamb, chops, loin, broiled, lean and fat	2.8 oz	235	0	22	16
lamb, chops, loin, broiled, lean only	2.3 oz	140	0	19	6
lamb, leg, roasted, lean only	2.6 oz	140	0	20	6
lamb, rib, roasted, lean only	2 oz	130	0	15	7
Pork					
cured, bacon, regular, cooked	3 slices	110	0	6	9
cured, ham, roasted, lean	2.4 oz	105	0	17	4
pork, luncheon meat, cooked ham, regular	2 slices	105	2	10	6
pork, luncheon meat, cooked ham, lean	2 slices	75	1	11	3
pork, chop loin, broiled, lean only	2.5 oz	165	0	23	8
pork, chop loin, pan-fried, lean only	2.4 oz	180	0	19	11
veal cutlet, braised, broiled	3 oz	185	0	23	9

Name	Amount	Calories	Carbohydrate (g)	Protein (g)	Fat (g)
Meat products					
bologna	2 slices	180	2	7	16
brown-and-serve sausage, cooked	1 link	50	0	2	5
frankfurter, cooked	1	145	1	5	13
salami, dry type	2 slices	85	1	5	7
Meals/Prepared Recipes					
beef and vegetable stew, homemade	1 cup	220	15	16	11
chicken à la king, homemade	1 cup	470	12	27	34
chicken chow mein, canned	1 cup	95	18	7	0
chicken potpie, homemade	1 piece	545	42	23	31
chili con carne w/beans, canned	1 cup	340	31	19	16
macaroni and cheese, canned	1 cup	230	26	9	10
quiche lorraine	1 slice	600	29	13	48
spaghetti, tomato sauce/cheese, homemade	1 cup	260	37	9	9
spaghetti, meatballs, tomato sauce, homemade	1 cup	330	39	19	12
cheeseburger, regular	1	300	28	15	15

Name	Amount	Calories	Carbohydrate (g)	Protein (g)	Fat (g)
enchilada	1	235	24	20	16
English muffin, egg, cheese, bacon	1 sandwich	360	31	18	18
fish sandwich, regular, w/cheese	1	420	39	16	23
hamburger, 4-oz. patty	1	245	28	12	11
pizza, cheese	1 slice	445	38	25	21
roast beef sandwich	1	290	39	15	9
taco	1	345	34	22	13
Nuts and Seeds					
almonds, slivered	1 cup	795	28	27	70
almonds, whole	1 oz	165	6	6	15
Brazil nuts	1 oz	185	4	4	19
cashew nuts, dry roasted, unsalted	1 oz	165	9	4	13
filberts (hazelnuts), chopped	1 oz	180	4	4	18
macadamia nuts, oil roasted, salted	1 oz	205	4	2	22
mixed nuts w/peanuts, oil roasted, unsalted	1 oz	175	6	5	16
peanuts, oil roasted, salted	1 oz	165	5	8	14

Name	Amount	Calories	Carbohydrate (g)	Protein (g)	Fat (g)
peanut butter	1 tbsp	95	3	5	8
pine nuts	1 oz	160	5	3	17
pistachio nuts	1 oz	165	7	6	14
sesame seeds	1 tbsp	45	1	2	4
sunflower seeds	1 oz	160	5	6	14
walnuts, English, pieces	1 oz	180	5	4	18
Poultry					
chicken, roasted, breast	3 oz	140	0	27	3
chicken, roasted, drumstick	1.6 oz	75	0	12	2
duck, roasted, flesh only	½ duck	445	0	52	25
turkey, roasted, dark meat	4 pieces	160	0	24	6
turkey, roasted, light meat	2 pieces	135	0	25	3
chicken, canned, boneless	5 oz	235	0	31	11
chicken frankfurter	1	115	3	6	9
Sauces					
cheese sauce w/milk, from mix	½ cup	153	13	8	8
hollandaise w/water, from mix	½ cup	120	7	3	10
white sauce w/milk, from mix	½ cup	120	10	5	6

Name	Amount	Calories	Carbohydrate (g)	Protein (g)	Fat (g)
barbecue sauce	1 tbsp	10	2	0	0
soy sauce	1 tbsp	10	2	2	0
beef gravy, canned	½ cup	65	6	4	3
chicken gravy, canned	½ cup	98	7	2	7
Soups					
bean with bacon soup, canned	1 cup	170	23	8	6
beef broth, bouillon, consommé, canned	1 cup	15	0	3	1
chicken noodle soup, canned	1 cup	75	9	4	2
clam chowder, Manhattan, canned	1 cup	80	12	4	2
clam chowder, New England, w/milk	1 cup	165	17	9	7
minestrone soup, canned	1 cup	80	11	4	3
pea, green, soup, canned	1 cup	165	27	9	3
tomato soup with milk, canned	1 cup	160	22	6	6
tomato soup w/ water, canned	1 cup	85	17	2	2
vegetable beef soup, canned	1 cup	80	10	6	2
vegetarian soup, canned	1 cup	70	12	2	2

Name	Amount	Calories	Carbohydrate (g)	Protein (g)	Fat (g)
chicken noodle soup, dehydrated, prepared	1 packet	40	6	2	1
onion soup, dehydrated, prepared	1 packet	20	4	1	0
Soy Foods					
soybeans, dry, cooked, drained	1 cup	235	19	20	10
miso	1 cup	470	65	29	13
tofu	1 piece	85	3	9	5
Sweets					
Candy, desserts, sugar					
caramels, plain or chocolate	1 oz	115	22	1	3
milk chocolate candy, plain	1 oz	145	16	2	9
fudge, chocolate, plain	1 oz	115	21	1	3
gumdrops	1 oz	100	25	0	0
hard candy	1 oz	110	28	0	0
jellybeans	1 oz	105	26	0	0
marshmallows	1 oz	90	23	1	0
gelatin dessert, prepared	½ cup	70	17	2	0
honey	1 tbsp	65	17	0	0

Name	Amount	Calories	Carbohydrate (g)	Protein (g)	Fat (g)
ice pop	1	70	18	0	0
jams and preserves	1 tbsp	55	14	0	0
pudding, chocolate, instant, from mix	½ cup	155	27	4	4
pudding, tapioca, from mix	½ cup	145	25	4	4
pudding, vanilla, from mix	½ cup	145	25	4	4
sugar, white, granulated	1 tbsp	45	12	0	0
sugar, white, granulated	1 packet	25	6	0	0
syrup, chocolate flavored, thin	2 tbsp	85	22	1	0
table syrup (corn and maple)	2 tbsp	122	32	0	0
Vegetables					
alfalfa seeds, sprouted, raw	1 cup	10	1	1	0
artichokes, globe, cooked	1	55	12	3	0
asparagus, cooked, cut	1 cup	45	8	5	1
snap beans, cooked	1 cup	45	10	2	0
bean sprouts, mung, cooked	1 cup	25	5	3	0
beets, cooked, diced	1 cup	55	11	2	0
beet greens, cooked	1 cup	40	8	4	0

Name	Amount	Calories	Carbohydrate (g)	Protein (g)	Fat (g)
black-eyed peas, cooked	1 cup	180	30	13	1
broccoli, raw	1 spear	40	8	4	1
broccoli, cooked	1 spear	50	10	5	1
broccoli, cooked	1 cup	45	9	5	0
brussels sprouts, cooked	1 cup	60	13	4	1
cabbage, raw	1 cup	15	4	1	0
cabbage, cooked	1 cup	30	7	1	0
carrots, raw, whole	1	30	7	1	0
carrots, raw, grated	1 cup	45	11	1	0
carrots, cooked	1 cup	70	16	2	0
cauliflower, raw	1 cup	25	5	2	0
cauliflower, cooked	1 cup	30	6	2	0
celery, raw	1 stalk	5	1	0	0
collards, cooked from raw	1 cup	25	5	2	0
collards, cooked from frozen	1 cup	60	12	5	1
corn, yellow, cooked	1 ear	85	19	3	1
corn, canned, whole kernel, white, no salt	1 cup	165	41	5	1

Name	Amount	Calories	Carbohydrate (g)	Protein (g)	Fat (g)
cucumber, w/peel	6 slices	5	1	0	0
eggplant, steamed	1 cup	25	6	1	0
endive, curly, raw	1 cup	10	2	1	0
kale, cooked	1 cup	40	7	2	1
kohlrabi, cooked	1 cup	50	11	3	0
lettuce, butter, raw	1 head	20	4	2	0
lettuce, crisp, raw	1 cup	5	1	1	0
lettuce, loose-leaf	1 cup	10	2	1	0
mushrooms, raw	1 cup	20	3	1	0
mushrooms, cooked	1 cup	40	8	3	1
okra pods, cooked	8	25	6	2	0
onions, raw, chopped	1 cup	55	12	2	0
onions, raw, sliced	1 cup	40	8	1	0
onions, raw, cooked	1 cup	60	13	2	0
onions, spring, raw	6	10	2	1	0
parsnips, cooked	1 cup	125	30	2	0
peas, edible pod, cooked	1 cup	65	11	5	0

Name	Amount	Calories	Carbohydrate (g)	Protein (g)	Fat (g)
peas, green, cooked	1 cup	125	23	8	0
peppers, red/green, raw	1	20	4	1	0
potatoes, baked, with skin	1	220	51	5	0
potatoes, baked, flesh only	1	145	34	3	0
potatoes, french-fried, frozen					
oven baked	10	110	17	2	4
fried	10	160	20	2	8
potatoes, mashed, dehydrated	1 cup	235	32	4	12
pumpkin, cooked from raw	1 cup	50	12	2	0
radishes, raw	4	5	1	0	0
sauerkraut, canned	1 cup	45	10	2	0
seaweed, kelp, raw	1 oz	10	3	0	0
spinach, raw	1 cup	10	2	2	0
spinach, cooked	1 cup	40	7	5	0
squash, summer, cooked	1 cup	35	8	2	1
squash, winter, baked	1 cup	80	18	2	1
sweet potatoes, baked, peeled	1	115	28	2	0

Name	Amount	Calories	Carbohydrate (g)	Protein (g)	Fat (g)
sweet potatoes, boiled, peeled	1	160	37	2	0
tomatoes, raw	1	25	5	1	0
tomatoes, canned, w/salt	1 cup	50	10	2	1
tomato juice, canned, w/o salt	1 cup	40	10	2	0
tomato paste, canned, w/o salt	1 cup	220	49	10	2
tomato puree, canned, w/o salt	1 cup	105	25	4	0
tomato sauce, canned, w/salt	1 cup	75	18	3	0
turnips, cooked, diced	1 cup	30	8	1	0
turnip greens, cooked	1 cup	30	6	2	0
vegetables, mixed, cooked	1 cup	105	24	5	0
water chestnuts, canned	1 cup	70	17	1	0
Miscellaneous Items					
Baking products, spices, vinegar					
baking powder, low sodium	1 tsp	5	1	0	0
catsup	1 tbsp	15	4	0	0
celery seed	1 tsp	10	1	0	1
chili powder	1 tsp	10	1	0	0
chocolate, bitter for baking	1 oz	145	8	3	15

Name	Amount	Calories	Carbohydrate (g)	Protein (g)	Fat (g)
cinnamon	1 tsp	5	2	0	0
coconut, raw	1 piece	160	7	1	15
coconut, raw, shredded	1 cup	285	12	3	27
curry powder	1 tsp	5	1	0	0
garlic powder	1 tsp	10	2	0	0
gelatin, dry	1 packet	25	0	6	0
mustard, prepared, yellow	1 tsp	5	0	0	0
olives, canned, green	4 medium	15	0	0	2
olives, canned, ripe, black	3 small	15	0	0	2
onion powder	1 tsp	5	2	0	0
oregano	1 tsp	5	1	0	0
paprika	1 tsp	5	1	0	0
pepper, black	1 tsp	5	1	0	0
pickles, cucumber, dill	1	5	1	0	0
salt	1 tsp	0	0	0	0
vinegar, cider	1 tbsp	0	1	0	0
yeast, brewer's, dry	1 tbsp	25	3	3	0

Shopping Lists

Vegetables

- Purchase enough greens to make salads for the week. (Option: prewashed bags contain enough lettuce for two to three large salads.)
- Purchase fresh vegetables that can be grilled or steamed. Frozen veggies are also an option, but contain fewer nutrients.

Protein/Meat

- eggs (one dozen)
- chicken breasts (bags contain up to twelve breasts)
- ground turkey
- precooked turkey breast (in deli section)
- cottage cheese, nonfat
- mozzarella cheese sticks, or low-fat varieties
- fish (fresh or frozen)

Fruit

- Seven pieces of favorite fruit (e.g., small apples)

Starches

- Oroweat Light bread
- Bran-a-Crisp bran crackers

Miscellaneous

- salad dressings (purchase two different varieties, two to three carbohydrates per serving *maximum*)
- seasonings and spices (for example, garlic powder, basil, pepper, mixed herb, Cajun)
- bouillon
- salt
- dill pickles (no sweet pickles!)
- nonstick cooking spray
- sugar-free gelatin (three to four packages)
- whipped topping
- drinks: water, diet soda, iced tea, low-carbohydrate diet drink mix (e g., Crystal Light)
- Twinfast shakes
- Ketostix

Bibliography

AMERICAN COLLEGE OF SPORTS MEDICINE. *ACSM Fitness Book,*
2d ed. Champaign, Ill.: American College of Sports Medicine, 1992.

ATKINS, R.C. *Dr. Atkins' New Carbohydrate Gram Counter.* New
York: M. Evans & Co., 1997.

BIRKETVEDT, G. S., J. FLORHOLMEN, J. SUNDSFJORD, B. OSTERUD,
D. DINGES, W. BILKER, and A. STUNKARD. "Behavioral and
Neuroendocrine Characteristics of the Night-Eating Syndrome." *Journal of the American Medical Association* 282
(1999): 657–63.

BRAY, G. "Health Hazards of Obesity." *Endocrinology and Metabolism Clinics of North America* 25, no. 4 (1996): 907–42.

CHEATHAM, B., AND C. R. KAHN. "Insulin Action and Insulin
Signaling Network." *Endocrine Review* 16 (1995): 117–42.

DESPRES, J. P., ET AL. "Hyperinsulinemia as an Independent Risk
Factor for Ischemic Heart Disease." *The New England Journal of Medicine* 334 (1996): 952–57.

DESPRES, J. P., B. LAMARCHE, P. MAURIEGE, B. CANTIN, P. J.
LUPIEN, AND G. R. DAGENAIS. "Risk Factors for Ischemic
Heart Disease: Is It Time to Measure Insulin?" *European
Heart Journal* 17 (1996): 1453–54.

EZRIN, C. "Childhood Diabetes." *University of Toronto Medical
Journal* 26 (1949): 233–39.

EZRIN, C., O. J. GODDEN, AND R. VOLPÉ. *Systematic Endocrinology,*
2d ed. New York: Harper & Row, 1979.

EZRIN, C., AND R. E. KOWALSKI. *The Type 2 Diabetes Diet Book,* 3d
ed. Los Angeles: Lowell House, 1999.

EZRIN, C., AND P. J. MOLONEY. "Resistance to Insulin Due to Neutralizing Antibodies." *Journal of Clinical Endocrinology and Metabolism* 19 (1959): 1055–68.

EZRIN, C., J. M. SALTER, M. A. OGRYZLO, AND C. H. BEST. "The Clinical and Metabolic Effects of Glucagon." *Canadian Medical Association Journal* 78 (1958): 96–98.

HELLER, R. F. *The Carbohydrate Addict's Gram Counter.* New York: Signet, 1993.

KERN, P. A., ET AL. "The Expression of Tumor Necrosis Factor in Human Adipose Tissue." *Journal of Clinical Investigation* 95 (1995): 2111–19.

KRAUS, B. *Calories and Carbohydrates,* 12th ed. New York: Penguin Books, 1997.

LONG, S. D., K. O'BRIEN, K. G. MAC DONALD, JR., N. LEGGET-FRAZIER, M. S. SWANSON, W. J. POUES, AND J. F. CARO. "Weight Loss in Severely Obese Subjects Prevents the Progression of Impaired Glucose Tolerance to Type II Diabetes." *Diabetes Care* 17 (1994): 372–75.

MCDONALD, A., A. NATOW, AND J. HESLIN. *Complete Book of Vitamins and Minerals.* Lincolnwood, Ill.: Publications International Ltd., 1994.

MOKDAD, A. H., ET AL. "The Spread of the Obesity Epidemic in the United States, 1991–1998." *Journal of the American Medical Association* 282 (1999): 1519–22.

MUST, A., ET AL. "The Disease Burden Associated with Overweight and Obesity." *Journal of the American Medical Association* 282 (1999): 1523–29.

NATIONAL TASK FORCE ON THE PREVENTION AND TREATMENT OF OBESITY. "Long-term Pharmacotherapy in the Management of Obesity." *Journal of the American Medical Association* 276 (1996): 1907–15.

NETZER, C. T. *Carbohydrate Gram Counter.* New York: Dell Publishing, 1994.

———. *The Complete Book of Food Counts.* New York: Dell Publishing, 1991.

PI-SUNYER, X. "Weight and Non-Insulin Dependent Diabetes Mellitus." *American Journal of Clinical Nutrition* 63, supplement 3 (1996): 4265–95.

PROCHASKA, J. D., J. C. NORCROSS, AND C. C. DI CLEMENTE. *Changing for Good: A Revolutionary Six-Stage Program for Overcoming Bad Habits and Moving Your Life Positively Forward.* New York: Avon, 1994.

SAFER, D. J. "Diet, Behavior Modification and Exercise: A Review of Obesity Treatments from Long-term Perspective." *Southern Medical Journal* 84 (1991): 1470–74.

STAHL, S. M., P. STANDOR, AND C. M. SHAPIRO. "Sleep Patterns in Depression and Anxiety: Theory and Pharmacological Effects." *Journal of Psychosomatic Research* supplement 1 (1994): 125–39.

SURATT, P. N., AND L. J. FINDLEY. "Driving with Sleep Apnea." *The New England Journal of Medicine* 340 (1999): 881–82.

UNITED STATES DEPARTMENT OF AGRICULTURE (USDA) Agricultural Research Service. *Nutrient Database for Standard Reference.* Release #12 (1998).

WILLIAMSON, D., AND L. PERRIN. "Behavioral Therapy for Obesity." *Endocrinology and Metabolism Clinics of North America* 24, no. 4 (1996): 943–55.

YOKE, M., AND L. GLADWIN. *A Guide to Personal Fitness Training.* Sherman Oaks, Calif.: Aerobics and Fitness Association of America, 1997.

Index

accident-prone persons, 26
acne, 25,
ACSM Fitness Book, 126
adrenocorticotropic hormone
    (ACTH), 142–43
alcohol consumption, 133, 36
American Diabetes Association,
    146
American Dietetic Association, 73
American Heart Association, 73
amino acids, 47
antidepressants, 46
appetite
    appetite control, 37, 38, 40–41
    excess insulin, 10
    drugs, 49
arthritis, 23
Asparagus Sesame Salad, 154
atherosclerosis, 60–61, 73
Atkins, Robert, 5–6

Beef
    Brisket with Chipotle Pepper
        Rub, 180
    Flank Steak, Grilled, 182
    Rolls, 180–81
    Satay, 182
    Wine and Herb, 184
Berson, Solomon, 144
beverage food list, 88
binge foods, 105, 108

blood pressure, high. *See* hyper-
    tension
body mass index (BMI), 26–27
body shape, 19
bread and crackers food list, 87

calcium supplement, 65
calories
    amount provided by diet, 64
    sources of, 63
cancer, and obesity, 21
carbohydrates
    complex, 72–73
    in diet, 63, 130–31
    intake for ketosis to occur,
        38–39, 42
    per serving (*See* food list, with
        carbohydrates per serving)
    restriction of, 11
    serotonin and, 12, 47
    simple, 72
    in stabilization phase, 129,
        130–31
cardiovascular disease, 60–61
cardiovascular exercise, 119–28
Cauliflower, Mushroom, and
    Onion Bake, 150–55
cereal food list, 87
Ceviche, Scallop, 174–75
Changing for Good (Prochaska),
    116

Cheeses, Three, with Tofu, 186
Chicken
    Almond, 155
    Cajun, 156
    Chinese Plum, 157
    Citrus, 158
    Grilled, with Citrus and Ginger, 159
    Italian, 159
    Kebabs, Ginger, 158
    Pesto, 160
    Pignolas and Spinach, 160–61
    Prosciutto, 161
    Ranch-Style, 161
    Rosemary and Garlic, 162
    with Sherry, Soy, and Ginger, 156
    Steamed with Vegetables, Spicy, 162–63
    with Sun-Dried Tomatoes, 156–57
    Taco, 163
    Three-Pepper, 163–64
children, obese, 32, 58
cholesterol levels, 72–73, 73
    gallbladder disease and, 20–21
    obesity and, 5–6
Cioppino, 167–68
cooking methods, 65
cortisol, 142, 143, 146
Cucumber and Tomato Salad, 151

diabetes, 20
    complications of, 57
    obesity and, 9, 18, 20, 57–61, 144–45
    Type 2, 57–61, 144–145

diabetes insipidus, 53
diary, dietary, 104–5, 106–7
diet, low-carbohydrate, low-calorie, 11
diet pills, 8
diuresis of recumbency, 54–55
diuretic drugs, 54
drink food list, 88

Eggplant, Pepper, and Tomato Salad, Spicy, 154–55
endocrinology, 141–47
    diabetes speciality and, 146–47
exercise, 119–128, 145
    aerobic, 11, 37, 119–28
    blood sugar levels and, 35
    cardiovascular, 119–28
    flexibility, 126–27
    importance of, 16
    obesity and, 5, 37
    staying motivated, 124–25
    target heart rate, 123–24
    water retention and, 52
    weight training, 125–26
exercise log, 128

family, 108–109, 115
fat, stored, 36–38
    as energy source, 11, 15
    insulin and, 143
    insulin resistance and, 145
    loss of, 39, 40
fats, dietary, 133–36
    calories in, 133
    functions of, 73
    monounsaturated, 73, 133
    need for, 73

polyunsaturated, 73, 133
reduction of, 6
restriction of, 39
saturated, 73, 133
types of, 73
fatty acids, 35, 36, 63, 133
fiber, dietary, 72–73, 130
Fish
    Catfish, BBQ, 166–67
    Flounder, Spinach–Stuffed,
        with Mushrooms and Feta
        Cheese, 176–77
    Halibut Brochettes, 170
    Mahi-Mahi, Tamari, 178–79
    Mahi-Mahi Stuffed with
        Veggies, 171
    Red Snapper Victoria, 172–73
    Salmon, Poached, with
        Vegetables, 171–72
    Salmon, with Cabernet Sauce,
        173–74
    Salmon, with Dill and Leeks en
        Papillote, 174
    Sole, Poached with Italian
        Vegetables, 172
    Sole, with Mustard and Dill, 176
    Swordfish, Baked, with Red
        Peppers and Mushrooms,
        166
    Swordfish, Grilled, with Red
        Pepper Salsa, 169
    Swordfish, in Chardonnay
        Sauce, 177
    Swordfish, Kebabs, 178
    Tuna, with Lemon and Sorrel,
        179
flexibility, 126–27

fluid retention. *See* water retention
food composition tables, 189–221
food list, with carbohydrates per
        serving and recommended
        serving size, 84–89
    bread, crackers, cereals, grains,
        and pastas, 87
    drinks, 88
    free foods, 87–88
    fruits, 86
    protein, 85
    sweets, 89
    vegetables, 85–86, 87, 89
food shopping lists, 223–24
free foods, 87–88
friends, 109–10, 115
fruits
    food list, 86, 87
    during stabilization phase, 130

gallbladder disease, 20–21
Gazpacho, 152
genetic factors, 34
grain food list, 87
Green Beans with Pancetta Bacon,
        152–153

habits, changing, 116
hemoglobin A1C, 60
herbal remedies for obesity, 8
high-density lipoproteins
        (HDLs), 61
high-protein diets, 63–64
holiday eating tips, 110–11,
        112–14
hyperinsulinemia, 60, 61, 144–45,
        147

hyperinsulinism, 19, 35, 39, 147
hyperlipidemia, 19
hypertension, 18–20, 60, 61
hypoglycemia, 47

infertility, 22–23
insulin
    dangers to obese, 5
    function of, 9, 143
    metabolism and, 9–11, 143
    role of, 9–11
    TNF-alpha and, 37, 144–45
    triglycerides and, 36
insulin control, 13–14, 33
Insulin Control Diet, 3–4
    calories eaten on, 64
    carbohydrate restriction, 64,
        72
    effects of, 39, 40–41
    expected weight loss on, 39
    initial weight-loss phase,
        83–101
    key components, 14
    maintenance phase,
        131–32, 133
    as panacea, 14
    protein requirement, 63, 65
    salt requirement, 51, 65
    stabilization phase, 129–31,
        136–39
    water intake, 72, 130
    weight-loss phase, 65–67, 72
insulin resistance, 57–58
    in obesity, 10–11, 57–58,
        143–145
    TNF-alpha and, 10, 58
    weight gain and, 10–11

Jenny Craig program, 7
journal, dietary, 104–5, 106–7,
    131, 136, 137

Kebabs
    Ginger Chicken, 158
    Swordfish, 178
ketoacidosis, diabetic, 36
ketones, testing for, 38, 41, 42–44,
    64, 130
ketosis, 35–44
    carbohydrate intake and, 36,
        38–44
    defined, 14, 35
    Insulin Control Diet and, 6
    metabolic trap of obesity and,
        35
    pregnancy and, 41–42
    safety of, 6
    during stabilization phase, 130
Ketostix (Ames Company), 38, 41,
    130
    use of, 42–44
kidneys, 64
Kowalski, Robert, 61
Kraus, Barbara, 89

leptin, 34, 37
lifestyle, 60, 119
Lindora program, 7–8
liver function, 21–22
low-carbohydrate diet, 11
    ketosis and, 36, 37, 38–44
low-density lipoproteins (LDLs), 61

maintenance phase of program,
    131–32, 133

caloric intake, 132
meal plans
for weight-loss phase, 65, 83–84
menus
weight-loss phase, initial,
89–101
Metabolic Trap of Obesity, 10–11
ketosis as key to unlocking, 35
Metabolic Trap of Obesity, and
ketosis, 42
metabolism
serotonin and, 11–13
milk products, 65
minerals, 74
sources and functions, 77–78
supplements, 65, 74
Moloney, Peter, 143–44
motivation, 124–25
muscle tissue, 40, 41
Mushrooms, Herbed, 153

Netzer, Corinne T., 89
NutriSystem program, 7
nutrition, 74–81
basics of, 71–81
recommended dietary
allowances (RDA), 74, 79–81
nuts, 133, 135

obesity, 4–8
beginnings of, 4–5
defined, 4
diabetes and, 9, 57–61
diet pills and, 8
evolution of, 33–34
genetic factors and, 34
herbal remedies, 8

insulin resistance and, 10–11,
57–58, 143–145
leptin and, 37
massive, 26, 28
medical risks of, 17–28, 32
Metabolic Trap of Obesity, 42
statistics, 31–32
traditional treatments, 5–8
Type 2 diabetes and, 57–61,
144–145
weight-loss programs and, 6–8
Opti-Fast program, 6–7
osteoarthritis, 23

pancreatitis, 18
pasta food list, 87
physicians, 49, 50, 63
consultation with, 66–67, 128
endocrinologists and diabetes
specialists, 146–47
Pima Indians, 34
pituitary gland, 141, 142
Pork
Brochettes, Rosemary, 181
Loin, Island, 183
Loin, Spanish, 183
poultry recipes, 155–65
prediabetic persons, 58
pregnancy, caution regarding
ketosis, 41–42
Prochaska, James, 116
protein, dietary, 39, 40, 41, 47
amount required, 63–64
food list, 85
during stabilization phase,
130, 131, 136, 137, 138
Prozac, 46, 48

recipes, 149–87
recommended dietary allowances
    (RDA), 74, 79–81
restaurant dining, 111–12
rewarding self, 115–17

Salsa, 169
salt, 37–38, 43, 44, 51, 65, 101
    required intake, 51
Seafood, 166–79. *See also* Fish
    Cioppino, 167–68
    Scallop Ceviche, 174–75
    Scallops, Grilled, with
        Portabella Mushrooms
        and Feta Cheese, 168–69
    Shrimp, Hot, 170
    Shrimp Mediterranean, 175–76
selective serotonin reuptake
    inhibitors (SSRIs), 45, 48, 49
serotonin, 26, 45–50
    carbohydrates and, 12, 26, 47
    control of, 13, 33
    excess, 48–49
    metabolism and, 11–13
    replenishment of, 12, 13, 16
    sleep and, 13
    stress and, 12–13, 46
    trazodone and, 13
shopping lists, 223–24
sibutramine, 49
skin disorders, 25
sleep, 12–13
    serotonin and, 12, 45–46
sleep apnea, 24
sodium. *See* salt
stabilization phase of program,
    129–31, 136–39

stevia, 89
Stir-Fry
    Tofu and Mixed Vegetable, 186
    Tofu and Portabello, 185
stress
    fluid retention and, 52
    serotonin and, 12–13, 46
support, emotional, 24, 108–11
    for exercising, 124
    strategies, 103–17
sweeteners, 89
sweets food list, 88

target heart rate, 123–24
thyroid gland, 141–42
TNF-alpha. *See* tumor necrosis
    factor alpha
Tofu
    Curry Seasoned, 184–85
    and Mixed Vegetable Stir-Fry,
        186
    and Portabello Stir–Fry, 185
    with Three Cheeses, 186–87
trazodone, 13, 20, 23, 24, 25, 46, 48,
    49, 50
trigger foods, 105, 108
triglycerides, 16, 17, 35, 61
tryptophan, 46, 47
tumor necrosis factor alpha (TNF-
    alpha), 10, 37, 58, 144–45
Turkey
    Piccata, 164–65
    Roll-Ups, 165
    Tex-Mex, 164

vegetables, 65, 130, 136
    food list, 85–86, 87

low-carbohydrate, food list,
85–86, 89
recipes, 150–55
starchy, food list, 87
virilizing adrenal hyperplasia, 142,
143, 146–47
vitamins, 74
fat-soluble, 73
sources and functions, 75–76
supplements, 65, 74

water, 44, 65
functions in body, 71–72
recommended intake, 72, 130
water retention, 37–38, 39, 43, 44,
51–55, 130
brain and, 54
causes, 52

urination and, 54–55
weight charts, 28, 29
weight-loss phase of program,
65–67
daily meal plan, 83–84
food list, with carbohydrate
per serving, 84–89
menus, 1000 calories per day,
89–101
when to end, 129–30
weight-loss programs, popular/
traditional, 6–8, 9
weight training, 125–26
Weight Watchers, 7

Yalow, Rosalyn, 144

Zucchini, Garlic, 152